Great Medical Discoveries

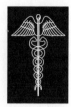

Heart Transplants

by Nancy Hoffman

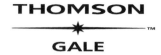

On cover: A team of doctors performs a heart transplant.

© 2003 by Lucent Books. Lucent Books is an imprint of The Gale Group, Inc.,
a division of Thomson Learning, Inc.

Lucent Books® and Thomson Learning™ are trademarks used herein under license.

For more information, contact
Lucent Books
27500 Drake Rd.
Farmington Hills, MI 48331-3535
Or you can visit our Internet site at www.gale.com

LIBRARY OF CONGRESS CATALOGING-IN-PUBLICATION DATA

Hoffman, Nancy, 1955—
    Heart transplants / by Nancy Hoffman.
        p. cm. — (Great medical discoveries)
Includes bibliographical references and index.
Summary: Discusses the history of man's knowledge of the heart, early
heart surgery, and the results, possible complications, costs, and
future of heart transplants.
    ISBN 1-56006-929-5 (hbk. : alk. paper)
    1. Heart—Transplantation—Juvenile literature [1. Heart—Transplantation.
2. Transplantation of organs, tissues, etc.] I.Title. II. Series
    RD598.35.T7 H65 2003
    617.4'120592--dc21   2002011050

Printed in the United States of America

CONTENTS

FOREWORD

Throughout history, people have struggled to understand and conquer the diseases and physical ailments that plague us. Once in a while, a discovery has changed the course of medicine, and sometimes, the course of history itself. The stories of these discoveries have many elements in common—accidental findings, sudden insights, human dedication, and, most of all, powerful results. Many illnesses that in the past were essentially a death warrant for their sufferers are today curable or even virtually extinct. And exciting new directions in medicine promise a future in which the building blocks of human life itself—the genes—may be manipulated and altered to restore health or to prevent disease from occurring in the first place.

It has been said that an insight is simply a re-arrangement of already-known facts, and, as often as not, these great medical discoveries have resulted partly from a reexamination of earlier efforts in light of new knowledge. Nineteenth-century monk Gregor Mendel experimented with pea plants for years, quietly unlocking the mysteries of genetics. However, the importance of his findings went unnoticed until three separate scientists, studying cell division with a newly improved invention called a microscope, rediscovered his work decades after his death. French doctor Jean-Antoine Villemin's experiments with rabbits proved that tuberculosis was contagious, but his conclusions were politely ignored by the medical community until another doctor, Robert Koch of Germany, discovered the exact culprit—the tubercle bacillus germ—years later.

Accident, too, has played a part in some medical discoveries. Because the tuberculosis germ does not stain with dye as easily as other bacteria, Koch was able to see it only after he had let a treated slide sit far longer than he intended. An unwanted speck of mold led Englishman Alexander Fleming to recognize the bacteria-killing qualities of the penicillium fungi, ushering in the era of antibiotic "miracle drugs."

That researchers sometimes benefited from fortuitous accidents does not mean that they were bumbling amateurs who relied solely on luck. They were dedicated scientists whose work created the conditions under which such lucky events could occur; many sacrificed years of their lives to observation and experimentation. Sometimes the price they paid was higher. Rene Launnec, who invented the stethoscope to help him study the effects of tuberculosis, himself succumbed to the disease.

And humanity has benefited from these scientists' efforts. The formerly terrifying disease of smallpox has been eliminated from the face of the earth—the only case of the complete conquest of a once deadly disease. Tuberculosis, perhaps the oldest disease known to humanity and certainly one of its most prolific killers, has been essentially wiped out in some parts of the world. Genetically engineered insulin is a godsend to countless diabetics who are allergic to the animal insulin that has traditionally been used to help them.

Despite such triumphs there are few unequivocal success stories in the history of great medical discoveries. New strains of tuberculosis are proving to be resistant to the antibiotics originally developed to treat them, raising the specter of a resurgence of the disease that has killed 2 billion people over the course of human history. But medical research continues on numerous fronts and will no doubt lead to still undreamed-of advancements in the future.

Each volume in the Great Medical Discoveries series tells the story of one great medical breakthrough—the first gropings for understanding, the pieces that came together and how, and the immediate and longer-term results. Part science and part social history, the series explains some of the key findings that have shaped modern medicine and relieved untold human suffering. Numerous primary and secondary source quotations enhance the text and bring to life all the drama of scientific discovery. Sidebars highlight personalities and convey personal stories. The series also discusses the future of each medical discovery—a future in which vaccines may guard against AIDS, gene therapy may eliminate cancer, and other, as yet unimagined, treatments may become commonplace.

INTRODUCTION

Heartfelt Changes

The human heart, long considered the body's emotional center, is still associated with feelings of love, the soul, and the spirit. The Greek philosopher Aristotle believed it to be the seat of sensation and thought, so important to life itself that it never suffered disease. Hippocrates, known as the father of medicine, believed any wound to the heart was fatal.

Today, it is understood that Aristotle and Hippocrates were wrong. Hearts do suffer disease. In fact, heart disease is the number one killer of Americans—according to the American Heart Association, one in every five deaths in the United States is due to heart disease. That is the bad news. The good news is that the heart is much more resilient than ancient doctors believed. It is not only capable of surviving a wound but of being cut open, repaired, and sewn back up, and severely diseased or damaged hearts can be replaced with healthy ones or even man-made hearts.

For those whose weak hearts have put them on the verge of death, heart transplantation is the cure of last resort. Many heart transplant recipients today live longer and with more vitality than some of those who underwent less serious heart operations in the early days of cardiac surgery.

Once heart surgery became a reality, heart transplantation was only decades away. Such rapid progress was propelled by innovative and sometimes brash surgeons and courageous patients. But the road to such progress had many obstacles.

A Remarkable Organ

The heart has long been thought of as much more than what physicians and scientists know it to be today—a highly efficient pump. Yet in that capacity the heart is remarkable. At only about the size of a human fist and weighing approximately three-quarters of a pound, the heart pumps blood through sixty thousand miles of blood vessels, a distance that is more than twice around the planet Earth, to reach all of the tissues in the human body. Together that network of blood vessels and the heart make up the human cardiovascular system.

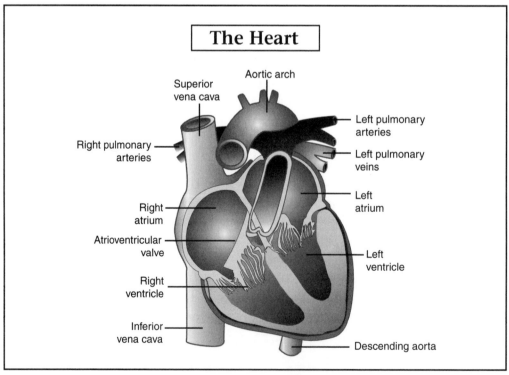

The Heart

A healthy adult's heart beats sixty times every minute, more than eighty-six thousand times each day, and over 2 billion times in an average lifetime. It pumps three ounces of blood with each beat, five and one-half quarts every minute, and over two thousand gallons a day.

The heart is much more than an efficient machine. It is affected by emotions. It beats faster when people are scared, excited, or angry, slower when people are relaxed. So perhaps it is not so difficult to understand why, throughout history, it has been thought to be not just a reactor to feelings but also the source of them.

Until the twentieth century, superstitions, emotions, and beliefs surrounding the heart both drove and delayed scientific knowledge and medical discoveries about it. Heart, or cardiac, surgery was the last frontier to be explored by surgeons.

By Accident

Christian Albert Theodor Billroth was a well-known and well-respected German surgeon, credited with being the founder of abdominal surgery. In the early 1880s, he declared, "Any surgeon who wished to preserve the respect of his colleagues would never attempt to suture the heart."[1] That remark stuck, and only the most courageous of surgeons would attempt work on the human heart.

More often than not, those surgeons who did operate on the heart did so by accident. After opening the chest and suturing all the wounds they could find, their patients were still bleeding. The only conclusion physicians could come to was that there were wounds penetrating the protective layer surrounding the heart and the heart itself. There was no way to view the inner chambers of the heart, so surgeons who worked on the heart were operating blindly. The only way to stop the bleeding and save the patient was to feel around and within the heart for the wound and sew it shut. This was the beginning of cardiac surgery. It would be some time before cardiac surgery was done on a regular basis. It was not until World War I and World War II that surgeons gained experience operating on the heart.

Fantastic Methods

By the time the first heart transplant was performed, surgeons had developed machines to keep patients alive while they opened up and examined diseased hearts to see what was wrong inside. In the decade and a half between "open" heart surgery and the first heart transplant, research surgeons had studied the possibility of what was thought of as the ultimate heart operation. As it happened, that first transplant did not occur in the United States, where the field of cardiac surgery was booming; rather, it took place halfway around the world, in Cape Town, South Africa.

To be the first surgeon to perform the operation, Dr. Christiaan Barnard had to find a patient who could stay alive long enough for the surgery and a family willing to donate the heart of their dying or brain-dead loved one for an experimental operation that might save a life. Timing was crucial; the necessary elements had to come together perfectly in order for Barnard to attempt such a feat.

On the morning of the operation, Barnard had his doubts:

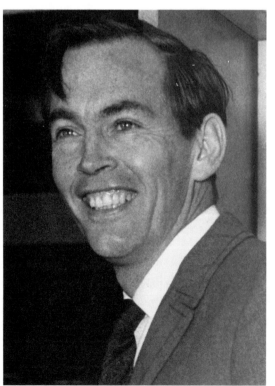

South African surgeon Dr. Christiaan Barnard was the first man to successfully perform a heart transplant.

I wanted to turn back, but there was no turning. Two people—a girl and a man—were now being moved into adjacent theaters [operating rooms]. Both of them had living hearts that could not continue to beat for much longer. We were approaching the moment when there would be nothing else to do other than cut out both their hearts, and place one of them—the girl's—within an empty chest of the man who would otherwise never leave the operating table alive.[2]

Barnard had more in common with all the cardiac surgeons who came before him and many who came after him than perhaps he realized: Between two dying patients, he could save only one life.

Chapter 1

To Hold and Heal a Human Heart

Heart surgery was not even attempted before the late 1800s—long after surgery on other human organs had been performed. Heart wounds were almost universally considered fatal. Lacking any effective treatment, most people with heart wounds simply died.

The medical community did not recognize the need for heart surgery, much less heart transplants, until surgeons developed the skills to perform heart surgery. A few doctors faced situations in which the only way to save a patient's life was to try something that had never been done before—surgery on a beating human heart. Those early heart surgeons were courageous people who risked failure and ridicule by taking a chance to help patients who tenaciously hung on to life. Such was the case with the first operation performed inside a human heart in Germany in 1896.

The Heart Kept Beating

At 7 A.M. on September 9, 1896, Dr. Louis Rehn arrived at Frankfurt City Hospital. Rehn was known as an innovative and daring pioneer among German surgeons. His patient was Wilhelm Justus, a young gardener's assistant, who had been brought to the hospital two days earlier by a policeman patrolling a city park.

Justus had been in a tavern fight and was fleeing assailants when he ran into the dark park. Drunk and tired, Justus staggered and stumbled. As he pulled himself up, an unknown assailant attacked him from behind, stabbing him several times in the chest with a knife. When Justus arrived at the hospital, he was slowly bleeding to death.

Hospital doctors held little hope for Justus to survive—in fact they did not expect him to live long enough for Rehn, head of the hospital's surgical division, to examine him.

During the examination, Rehn found a stab wound to Justus's pericardium (the protective sac surrounding the heart). The prevailing opinion of physicians at that time was that suturing heart wounds was unnecessary because either the wound itself or a surgical cut to the heart would most likely kill the patient. However, Rehn had seen evidence that this was not true. Rehn recalled reading about successful experimental cardiac surgery performed on rabbits and dogs. Defying the expert medical opinion of the time, Rehn decided to try to save Justus's life. To do so, Rehn would have to see, feel, and hold a living heart in his hands. The operation began at 7:27 A.M.

After Justus was given anesthesia, Rehn made an incision in his patient's chest five and one-half inches long. He then cut Justus's fifth rib and folded it inward so he could see Justus's heart and examine his wounds. Blood flooded the patient's open chest. Rehn stuck his finger through the wound to see how deep it was. Blood spilled out, and air entered the open cavity. Justus's lung collapsed, and Rehn told the anesthetist to stop anesthesia.

Rehn had difficulty gripping the pericardium, so he cut farther into it. Peering into Justus's chest, Rehn found another wound, one-half inch long, in the middle of the wall of the right ventricle. Rehn put his finger on the wound, and the bleeding stopped.

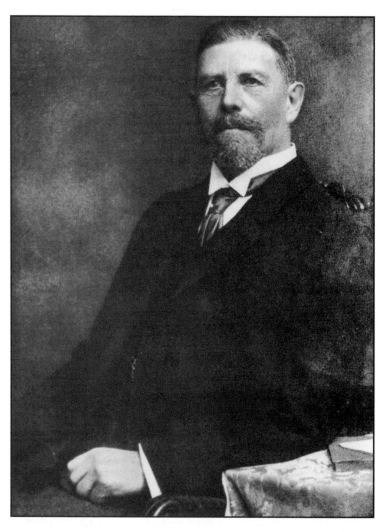

Dr. Louis Rehn proved the benefits of cardiac surgery after performing a daring heart operation.

An assistant handed Rehn a fine needle with a silk thread. While he continued to cover the wound in Justus's heart, Rehn began to stitch it closed. It was difficult because the heart kept beating. Rehn tied the first knot, then the second, and finally the last one. The bleeding stopped, and Justus's heart kept beating.

Rehn then rinsed out the pericardium and the chest cavity, clearing away the blood. He drained the pericardium, replaced the rib, and finally closed the external wound. A few weeks later, Wilhelm Justus was out of danger and well on his way to a full recovery.

What Rehn did after the operation was just as important as the operation itself. A year after the surgery on Justus, Rehn spoke about this pioneering heart operation at a surgeons' congress in Berlin. He ended his speech with these words: "The possibility of performing cardiac suture certainly can no longer be doubted . . . I trust that his case will not remain a mere curiosity, but that it will stimulate further work in the field of cardiac surgery, transforming this new field into a life-saving branch of our profession."[3]

Louis Rehn had opened the door for other surgeons who would follow him to explore the possibilities of heart surgery.

War and Traveling Bullets

While Rehn's ideas were influential, relatively few heart surgeries were actually attempted until World War I left multitudes of men wounded. Most surgeons were afraid of the difficulties of heart surgery. Cutting into an open chest would let air into the pleural, or lung, cavity, which could make breathing impossible for the patient. This had been a problem for Rehn, who had to contend with one of Justus's lungs collapsing. Rehn had been fortunate; his patient was still able to breathe for the duration of the operation.

At the beginning of World War I, physicians considered heart surgery too great a risk for the patient—not enough was known about how the heart would respond to surgery. However, as the war progressed, soldiers' wounds became more complicated and less clean. For physicians, the straight, clean stab wounds caused by the crimes and accidents of civilian life were replaced by muddy, jagged bullet and shrapnel fragment wounds to the pericardium and the heart muscle. These wounds often caused painful bruising and serious cuts, or lacerations, which led to infection. Because these soldiers' wounds became infected, military surgeons were forced to open the chest and operate in order to drain the pus. If this was not done, the infection could easily kill the patient.

The wounded continued to flood army hospitals; more and more heart surgery was done to avoid infection, but little was recorded. *The History of the Great War Medical Services: Surgery of the War* reported, "No doubt a considerable number of operations have been performed in which rents [tears] in the pericardium were repaired, or retained foreign bodies removed, but unfortunately few records of these are available."[4]

Due to the sheer volume of wounded soldiers, most heart and other operations were as short and simple as possible. According to *The Medical Department of the United States Army in the World War*, "Early operations upon the heart and pericardium have been few because wounds affecting them are either promptly fatal or treated expectantly [using simple well-known procedures]. Such injuries as are disclosed by operation are easily remedied as they require little more than simply suturing."[5]

Although most World War I soldiers wounded in the heart died on the battlefield, many who did survive had evidence of their wounds show up months, sometimes years, later. Often, bullets and pieces of shrapnel lost in the body would migrate from organ to organ, sometimes being carried in the bloodstream. Bullets from old wounds created new wounds, which led to new operations. Fortunately, X-ray machines, developed at the end of the nineteenth century, helped surgeons find the source of most bullet wounds.

One particular case demonstrates just how long a man could live between being wounded and having surgery. A French soldier wounded at the battle of Bapaume on August 27, 1914, was taken prisoner by the Germans. His injuries did not seem serious at first. But six months later he suffered frequent heart attacks and a sensation of impending death. An X ray showed a bullet in his heart. In April 1917, he traveled to Paris and was put into the care of Dr. Henri Hartmann, who successfully operated on him. Hartmann removed the bullet from the right ventricle of his heart—more than two and one-half years after the bullet entered the soldier's body.

There were many cases of bullets entering soldiers' hearts through the ventricular cavity and then being carried out of the heart in the bloodstream into other parts of the body. In many cases the force of the bloodstream was quite strong. French surgeon Pierre Duval found a bullet "like an egg dancing on a jet of water,"[6] where the inferior, or lower, vena cava (the main vein returning blood to the heart) met with the left atrium of the heart. The operation to remove the bullet took just thirty-five minutes, and the patient went on to a quick and full recovery.

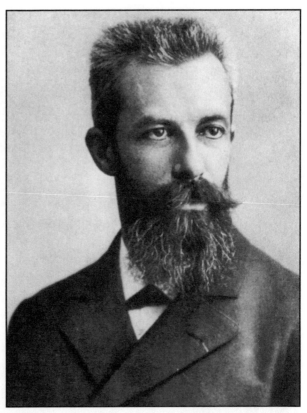

Henri Hartmann was among the doctors who attempted cardiac surgery during World War I.

While many bullets were removed from World War I soldiers, many remained. "It is a common experience that bullets frequently lodge in the tissue and induce neither local nor general infection until attempts for removal are made,"[7] wrote British surgeon Charles Ballance in the well-known medical journal *The Lancet*. Some surgeons did not feel competent to operate; others felt that removing the foreign bodies would only cause additional health problems for their patients. As late as 1947, Jerome R. Head, a surgeon in Chicago who had examined many World War I veterans, found many of his patients still had bullets and other foreign bodies left in their chests. Head said that he had seen "only two in whom these were causing trouble."[8]

World War II and Pioneering Surgeons

After gaining surgical experience during World War I, surgeons gained confidence in treating heart wounds by means of operating inside an open chest. By the time World War II erupted in Europe, many more doctors were proficient in the art of cardiac surgery. Some even became pioneers, pushing heart surgery to the point where heart transplantation could be considered a viable option for the future.

In 1942, the U.S. Army's medical manual included directions for dealing with heart wounds. The first of these instructions was to aspirate, or suction out, blood from the pericardium; the second was to repeat the first procedure if necessary; and the final step was to operate if steps one and two failed to work. The army's instructions proved to be good ones by a study on nonoperative treatment for cardiac tamponade—a condition in which pressure from fluid makes the pericardium so tight around

A doctor and two aides treat a wounded man during World War II. By this time, doctors were able to save many soldiers who suffered wounds to the heart.

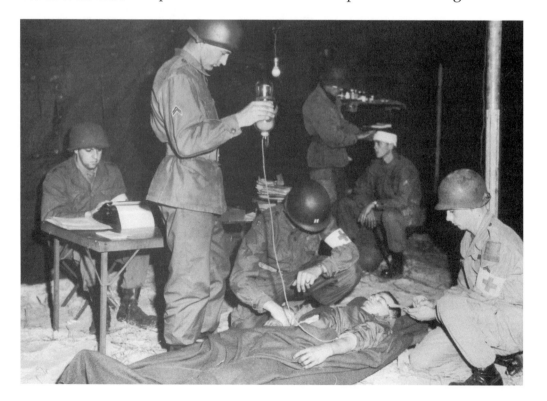

the heart that the heart cannot expand normally to pump blood. The study, done by Alfred Blalock and Mark Ravitch at Johns Hopkins (a prestigious U.S. medical school and hospital), marked the beginning of modern treatment for heart wounds. Blalock and Ravitch found it was often better to delay surgery to see if the wound might heal itself and to build up the strength of the patient so he or she could fight infection if an operation were performed. As a result of the U.S. Army's adopting this method of treatment, far more soldiers survived heart wounds in World War II than in World War I.

While cardiac surgery techniques progressed, so did other areas of medicine. Before and during World War II, the Allies stockpiled blood through donor campaigns in Europe and the United States. At this time, plasma was successfully separated from blood and used as a blood substitute. Plasma is the part of blood that remains after all the cells have been removed. Plasma does not have to be typed—any patient can safely receive the plasma of any donor—and it can be stored longer and survives rougher handling than whole blood. The coordinated efforts to collect blood and produce plasma developed into an adequate blood-transfusion service. Blood transfusions are essential to strengthen the wounded before cardiac surgery and to prevent them from going into shock from loss of blood.

Researchers also developed infection-fighting drugs during World War II. In 1940 the first antibiotic, penicillin, was manufactured for clinical use. Penicillin helps fight disease-causing bacteria. Later, sulfonamides were used similarly. Dealing more aggressively with infection allows for a better recovery from the trauma of cardiac surgery. Although infection is still a problem for surgeons, new and better antibiotics have ensured better patient recovery. All of these developments set the stage for advancement in heart surgery and better treatment of soldiers wounded in battle.

Soldiers wounded in World War II were evacuated to base camps and then moved to forward hospitals, which were special centers set up for those wounded in the chest. It was at the forward hospitals that new cardiac surgery methods were being developed by innovative and observant surgeons. One of the most successful of these surgeons was Dwight Harken of Boston. A skillful surgeon who loved cardiac surgery, Harken learned those new methods quickly. As a U.S. Army officer working in London, Harken removed 134 missiles (what bullet and shrapnel particles were routinely called) from the hearts of wounded soldiers without losing a single patient.

In 1945, a *New York Times* reporter described Harken as "a sandy-red-haired six-foot Bostonian who looked only slightly older than the age of his average case."[9] Harken's youthful enthusiasm for his work was infectious, and he quickly became a leader in the field of cardiac surgery. He also appreciated teamwork. Harken's attitude and that of other surgeons like him created an atmosphere of cooperation in the military medical community. Often Harken and those who worked with him would leave the hospital at night and go act as consultants elsewhere. "We were young and vigorous and didn't worry about sleeping," said Harken. "The next morning after these trips, we'd just go back to work."[10]

During one particularly dramatic operation, Harken used his fingers and thumb to put pressure on the right ventricle of his patient's heart. He then worked for more than three minutes to dislodge a piece of shrapnel from inside the heart. Previously, surgeons would have avoided probing deeper inside the heart, fearing the patient would not survive the ordeal. Throughout the procedure, the soldier's heart continued to beat and maintain adequate blood pressure. Harken had proved the human heart could withstand much more in the operating arena than had earlier been believed. Anesthetist Charles Burstein said of

Prisoner Exchange

In wartime, it is not unusual for military doctors and surgeons to treat enemy prisoners of war. In fact it is often necessary to ensure the safety of soldiers captured behind enemy lines.

In Europe during World War II, two titans of surgery headed the wartime medical efforts for the Allies and the Germans. A. Tudor Edwards was considered by the British and much of the English-speaking world to be the father of thoracic (chest) surgery. Ernst Ferdinand Sauerbruch held that title in his native Germany and on the rest of the European continent.

Tudor Edwards disliked Sauerbruch long before the war. That was because Tudor Edwards had been passed over for foreigner Sauerbruch to treat the Prince of Wales when he was ill with a lung infection in 1935. Tudor Edwards never forgave nor forgot the incident.

Boston's Dwight Harken worked on Tudor Edwards's wartime medical team. Part of Harken's job was to help select chest-injured German prisoners to exchange for American prisoners. Germany's Sauerbruch selected the Americans. Harken grew to agree with Tudor Edwards's opinion of Sauerbruch. Harken claimed Sauerbruch "cheated" in choosing which wounded American prisoners to release. The released Americans were often so badly injured they did not survive the trip back to the United States. The Nazi doctor sent back irreparable paraplegics or amputees with chest wounds that could never be repaired, ignoring the humane principle of selecting those wounded who were most able to make the trip home. Harken also believed Sauerbruch ignored the Geneva covenant, which forbade the return to combat of exchanged prisoners. According to Harken, wounded German prisoners, well cared for by the Americans, seemed reluctant to be released back to their own side.

working with Harken, "We approached every operation with the expectation of success—and we did succeed."[11]

Harken was also one of the first to realize that only through an operation could a doctor be certain that a missile was not lodged in the heart. A bullet in the lung, not even in the pericardium, could sometimes move in time with the heartbeat, and its location could not be detected even by X ray. While Harken followed the army's suggestions concerning whether or not to operate, he admitted to being influenced in favor of surgery if there was any uncertainty or if the patient was in pain.

Harken learned all he could from the operations he performed. For instance, he realized that the heart worked best when it was not moved from its location in the body. A slight nudge by a surgeon's hand moving the organ out of place could disrupt heart rhythm. But he also learned a surgeon's fingers could work within the heart while it continued to pump blood throughout the body.

Harken relished teaching others what he had learned in surgery. Many young surgeons sought his guidance and thrived under his direction. One military surgeon decided to forgo a promotion just to work with Harken.

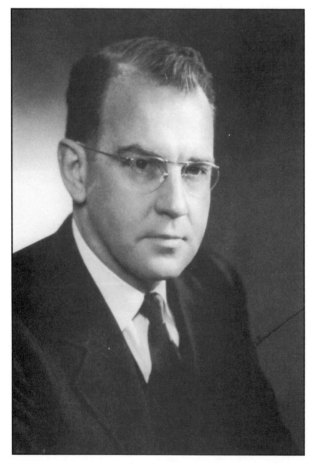

Dr. Dwight Harken's pioneering efforts in cardiac surgery earned him a reputation as a leader in his field.

Peacetime Progress

The experience surgeons gained and the spirit of teamwork that developed during World War II, the development of antibiotics, and the arrival of an adequate blood-transfusion service all contributed to the rapid growth of cardiac surgery. In fact, heart surgery progressed faster than any other medical field in the two decades following World War II.

Harken, like many of the surgeons he worked with, believed that what he learned during the war could also be applied to peacetime operations. Heart disease, rather than war wounds, soon became the focus of a heart surgeon's work. The progress made during World War II increased the understanding of the heart and gave doctors more ways to combat heart disease. The first area that physicians explored was congenital heart disease, which is the term for abnormalities present at birth such as holes in the heart or defective heart valves.

Before cardiac surgery existed, the medical profession had virtually ignored congenital heart defects. Doctors had difficulty diagnosing those defects until serious symptoms such as irregular heartbeat, shortness of breath, and extreme fatigue appeared. Little could be done to treat those symptoms, so patients were simply made as comfortable as possible. As more heart surgery was done, more was understood about congenital heart defects. And pioneering surgeons sought out ways to correct what was wrong.

Whether or not to treat a congenital birth defect surgically depended on the specific abnormality and its severity. Statistically, about eight babies in one thousand have a heart malformation. Some are mild, and in many cases the child outgrows the problem—the defect corrects itself as the child grows. For example, in most cases a hole in a child's heart closes by itself over time. However, other cases require an operation to correct the problem.

One condition that warrants an operation is coarctation, or constriction, of the aorta. This condition impedes blood flow from the heart. A child with this condition experiences increased blood pressure, which in time can become irreversible. Fifty percent of the babies born with this condition die in their first year of life if left untreated. In the 1940s, heart surgeons began experimenting on animals to find a way to correct congenital heart defects, including coarctation of the aorta.

After years of operating on laboratory dogs, Swedish surgeon Clarence Crafoord developed a method of removing the coarctation of the aorta. By cutting out the constricted area, Crafoord found he could suture together the remaining ends and restore the aorta to a normal width, allowing blood to flow freely through it. On October 19, 1944, in Stockholm, Sweden, Crafoord and Gustave Nylin successfully performed this procedure on a twelve-year-old boy. In June 1945, Robert Gross and Charles Hufnagel, both of Boston, performed a similar operation on a five-year-old boy. Unfortunately, the patient died. But a month later Gross and Hufnagel used the same technique to save the life of a twelve-year-old girl.

Crafoord and Gross developed the same procedure separately, but their method has survived the test of time; surgeons still use it today. The technique has saved and lengthened lives.

Curing Blue Babies

In the 1940s, other operations on congenital defects were more difficult because surgeons were operating blind. There was no way of keeping the patient's blood circulating and the patient breathing if the heart was cut open enough for the surgeon to see what he or she was doing. Surgeons just had to hunt around and find holes with their fingers and suture them without seeing them completely.

The fear of operating blind did not stop two doctors from developing an operation to save blue babies.

Congenital cyanotic heart disease is a condition in which blood from the two sides of the heart mixes. The result is unoxygenated, or blue, blood being pumped throughout the body. The patient is cyanosed, meaning the skin has a bluish discoloration. Several kinds of heart defects can cause this condition, the most common being Fallot's tetrad, a combination of four defects in the heart: a misplaced aorta, a hole between the two ventricles, a narrowing and thickening of the valve leading to the right ventricle, and a dilating and thickening of the valve leading from the right ventricle. Babies born with Fallot's tetrad, if untreated, rarely survived beyond their second birthday.

After a couple of years as director of the pediatric cardiac clinic at Johns Hopkins Hospital in Baltimore, Maryland, Helen Taussig noticed that some babies with Fallot's tetrad were healthier than others. She found the babies who were healthier had an additional defect, that of patent ductus. There is an artery in the heart that directs blood to the lungs of the fetus. At birth the artery normally closes, except in babies with patent ductus.

It was Taussig's initial observation that gave her the insight into the treatment of Fallot's tetrad. Taussig thought there might be a way to create patent ductus, or at least a bypass similar to it, in babies with Fallot's tetrad.

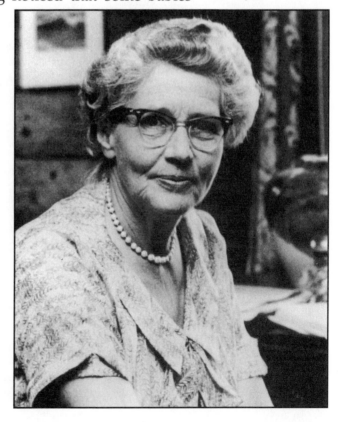

Helen Taussig helped develop a treatment for congenital heart disease after observing infants with cardiac birth defects.

This bypass would increase the blood supply to the lungs, thereby relieving most of the symptoms of cyanosis.

Taussig discussed her observations with Baltimore surgeon Alfred Blalock. Taussig's sharing her discovery with Blalock led to the development of a new surgical treatment for congenital heart disease. The two physicians experimented on laboratory animals and came up with a procedure in which they divided an arterial branch of the aorta and joined it to the pulmonary artery. On October 29, 1944, Blalock successfully operated on a fifteen-month-old girl.

The third operation of this kind by Blalock convinced Taussig that all her work had been worthwhile. The patient was what Taussig described as an "utterly miserable small six-year-old boy who had a red blood cell count of 10 million (twice normal) and was no longer able to walk." Taussig recalls that when Blalock removed the clamps from the aorta and pulmonary artery, anesthesiologist Dr. Merle Harmel cried, "He's a lovely color now!" When the boy woke up in the operating room, he asked Blalock if he could get up. From that moment on Taussig found the boy to be "a happy, active child."[12]

Attacking Mitral Stenosis

Not all diseases of the heart are present at birth; many heart problems are caused by other diseases. Rheumatic fever, an illness caused by certain bacteria, can seriously damage the valves of the heart and is almost always the cause of mitral stenosis.

Mitral stenosis is the most common form of heart disease and one of the cruelest in that it most often strikes once-healthy children and young adults. In mitral stenosis, a valve in the heart becomes tight or obstructed. In turn, not enough blood can flow into the left ventricle, causing the left ventricle to enlarge and back up or regurgitate blood into the lungs. All of this taxes the heart's ability to work normally. Surgery to correct this condition would seem only logical—in fact one was successfully performed in 1925 by British surgeon Henry Souttar. Souttar cut into the heart to reach the mitral valve. He was able to remove the obstruction with his finger, returning the valve to normal. Unfortunately, Souttar's success was considered a fluke, and the operation he performed unjustifiable, by the medical community of the time. Few doctors believed an obstruction could be removed so easily by a surgeon's finger so that in most cases Souttar's method would fail. All surgical efforts to combat mitral stenosis were abandoned until 1948.

On June 10, 1948, at Philadelphia General Hospital, a pioneering cardiac surgeon named Charles Bailey

Souttar Took a Chance to Save a Life

In her short life in the slums of London, Lily Hine had suffered from asthma, bronchitis, and rheumatic fever. By 1925, when she turned fifteen, she was skinny and miserable—even breathing was difficult. Lily also had a chronic cough and pain in her joints and limbs, the classic symptoms of mitral stenosis.

Cardiologist T.B. Layton had seen many patients like Lily, and he was convinced the girl could not survive six more months. As a last resort, Layton took her to Henry Souttar at London Hospital. The two men agreed that an innovative operation by Souttar was the girl's only chance.

On May 6, 1925, Souttar made a C-shaped incision in Lily's chest, bent back her ribs and exposed her heart. He made a half-inch incision in the heart so he could explore the mitral valve and clean out the obstruction, which he was able to do

with his finger. The girl's blood pressure fell to zero but her heart kept beating. There was a leak. Souttar found and repaired it. He thought the operation was over and withdrew his finger. Blood spurted out again. There was another leak. Quickly yet gently, Souttar repaired the second leak. The bleeding stopped, Lily's blood pressure went back to normal, and Souttar felt the valve opening and closing normally.

Lily recovered quickly after the surgery, having more energy than ever before. Unfortunately, a few years later she suffered more bouts of rheumatic fever and died in 1932.

In 1961, Dwight Harken wrote to Souttar asking why he never followed up his initial success. Souttar wrote back to Harken that the medical community's response to his surgery was less than enthusiastic. "In fact it is of no use to be ahead of one's time," Souttar concluded.

made two attempts to remove an obstruction in the mitral valve using the same method Souttar had. The first operation failed. The second, done only upon the insistence of the twenty-four-year-old patient, succeeded. The young woman was active and well for years afterwards.

Six days later, unaware of Bailey's success, Dwight Harken successfully performed virtually the same procedure. That same month Russell Brock in England also successfully operated on the mitral valve. All made the same discovery as Souttar independently of each other.

It had taken more than twenty years for Souttar's method to be appreciated and recognized as one of the turning points in cardiac surgery. Souttar's early success, and those of Bailey, Harken, and Brock a generation later, eventually led to other methods to combat valvular disease, including valve replacement.

Heart surgery was becoming more complex and more promising. Yet surgeons were still using their sense of touch to examine and repair the human heart. Finally, in the 1950s, it became possible to cut into a heart and expose its inner workings—the procedure known as open-heart surgery.

CHAPTER 2

Open-Heart Surgery

Cutting into a beating heart to heal it almost seems like a contradiction in terms. But for 1950s cardiac surgeons, open-heart surgery became the obvious next step in their battle against heart disease. In order to do this they would have to find a way not only to continue blood flow throughout the body but also to ensure that blood was oxygenated (mixed with oxygen). Pioneering surgeons tried out several methods for open-heart surgery.

The medical equipment and techniques used in a state-of-the-art operating room in 1954 would seem very out of date today. Nurses used two fingers on the inside of the patient's wrist and a wall clock with a large second hand to monitor pulse, glass thermometers to take temperatures, and blood pressure cuffs and stethoscopes to check blood pressure. Electrocardiogram machines to record heart rate and rhythm were available but seldom used. Other operating room machines such as electric suction pumps and generators often interfered with the electrocardiogram, rendering it inaccurate.

The newest anesthesia in 1954 was cyclopropane. Although safer than ether, it was highly inflammable. Doctors and nurses in operating rooms had to wear special shoes and could not wear silk or nylon for fear of static electricity creating a spark and causing the cyclopropane to explode.

Even with these limitations, cardiac surgery was considered a glamorous field on the verge of exciting developments. The news media began reporting on each new "unbelievable and fantastic" operation as if medical history was being made; in many cases, it was.

The seriousness of heart disease began to be recognized following World War II. At the same time, the American Heart Association (AHA) grew from a small group of cardiologists to the national agency in the heart field. The AHA became a major outlet for heart-related medical information and a powerful political lobbyist and fundraiser dedicated to fighting heart disease. In 1946, the AHA predicted 658,000 people would die from heart disease that year alone, while cancer would only claim the lives of 183,000. President Harry Truman called heart disease the nation's most challenging health problem. In 1950,

A team of doctors performs open-heart surgery in the 1950s. While comparatively primitive to modern medical science, cardiac surgery during this time yielded many discoveries.

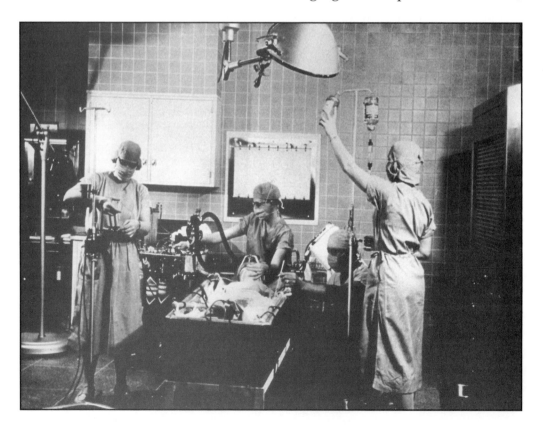

Truman proclaimed February as National Heart Month, saying, "Measures to cope with this threat are of immediate concern to every one of us."[13] By adopting the slogan "New Hope for Hearts," the AHA helped bring heart disease into the national spotlight. All the publicity and recognition eventually led to more money for research and more support for heart surgeons determined to pioneer new techniques.

Many heart surgeons were anxious for the new developments but frustrated with their limitations. The most renowned of these surgeons were innovative and willing to take risks some might call reckless. The competition between top heart surgeons was fierce—a race for every new development. And the first race was for a method or machine to sustain a patient's life during open-heart surgery.

Hypothermia

During World War II, the Nazis tried to determine how much cold the human body could tolerate, by experimenting on prisoners. What they discovered was that human beings could be cooled to low levels for a short period of time and then warmed up and survive without developing any major complications. It appeared that the bodily functions of humans, much like those of hibernating animals, were suspended when body temperature was lowered. Maverick heart surgeon Charles Bailey had read about the gruesome research and wondered if cold could reduce the demand on the heart to oxygenate blood long enough for open-heart surgery to be attempted.

Bailey, working at the Hahnemann Medical College and Hospital in Philadelphia, began experimenting on different methods of lowering the temperature of dogs. First he tried a cooling chamber and then a rubberized cooling blanket. By lowering the dog's temperature to just below 30 degrees Celsius (86 degrees Fahrenheit), Bailey found he could shut off the blood to the animal's heart for twelve minutes without hurting the dog. This

Antivivisectionists

Antivivisectionists are people who oppose animal research, especially experimentation involving pain or death for the animals. Medical researchers contend that lives are saved by such practice and that their research would be impossible without using animals. A strong antivivisection movement in Great Britain—having exerted pressure on British lawmakers since the time of Queen Victoria—stalled cardiac research there for years. While not as influential in the United States, they let their opinions be known, often shouting them at lab personnel and researchers.

A group of antivivisectionists did not like what was happening in the University of Minnesota research lab in Millard Hall. They worked to overturn Minnesota's law on animal experimentation. They also wrote angry notes to doctors and lab personnel. One letter writer called researchers savages. The antivivisectionists remembered a 1939 article in the Minneapolis Tribune about a dog-napping ring. Reportedly, thieves stole five hundred household pets and sold them to the University of Minnesota for $2.50 each.

Rumors of similar pet-snatching rings still abound in many communities today. But success usually results in support for research, and such was the case with the University of Minnesota Hospital's heart surgery program and its local newspaper. In a September 23, 1952 Minneapolis Tribune editorial entitled "14 Dogs Died So She and Other Children Have a Chance to Live," the writer stated: "One child at the price of fourteen dogs is a remarkable bargain any way you figure it. Minnesota should be proud that its laws enable its scientists to save human life this cheaply."

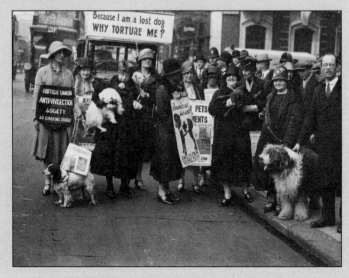

Dog lovers march in London in support of a 1925 antivivisection bill.

procedure allowed Bailey a few minutes to operate—
long enough to open the heart and repair a hole
between the heart's two upper chambers, a condition
referred to as atrial septal defect, or ASD. After a series
of tests on dogs, Bailey was ready to try an operation
on a human with ASD.

On August 29, 1952, he attempted the first open-
heart surgery on a thirty-year-old woman with a large
ASD. Bailey reduced her temperature to 27 degrees
Celsius (80 degrees Fahrenheit) and opened her heart.
The operation went well until he unclamped the vessels going into her heart; then her heart began beating
irregularly. Apparently, air bubbles had gotten into
the woman's arteries. She died on the operating table.

Just days later, surgeon F. John Lewis at University
Hospital in Minneapolis tried Bailey's technique on a
child with suspected ASD. Five-year-old Jacqueline
Johnson, the underweight daughter of traveling carni-
val workers, had been sick most of her life. Lewis
thought the experimental operation was the girl's
only chance for survival.

On September 2, 1952, Jacqueline's temperature
was lowered to 28 degrees Celsius (82 degrees
Fahrenheit). Her heart rhythm went from 120 to 60
beats per minute. Lewis cut through the wall of her
right atrium, and within four minutes he found the
hole and sutured it closed. (At normal temperature,
four minutes is the point at which oxygen-deprived
brain cells start to die.) Lewis closed the girl's heart
and then massaged it back to normal rhythm. Finally,
he closed her chest, and she was immersed in a tub of
warm water. The Minnesota surgeon had bought a
Farm Master watering trough from a Sears, Roebuck
catalog just for this occasion. Eleven days after the
operation, Jacqueline, the first successful open-heart
patient, went home healthy.

Lewis's success inspired many others. Soon after his
operation on Jacqueline Johnson, most major universities began developing their own open-heart programs.

But hypothermia had many disadvantages. It did not allow enough time for repairing more complicated heart defects. Lewis attempted surgery on patients with ventricular septal defect, or VSD. A VSD is a hole between the heart's lower two chambers that is difficult to get to surgically. He was unsuccessful, losing two patients, both of whom were children. While other surgeons joined in the competition to be the first to repair VSDs and other more complicated conditions, Lewis lost interest in open-heart surgery—he just could not bear losing any more young patients.

Cross Circulation

In 1953, Morley Cohen, a surgeon who ran the research lab for Lewis at the University of Minnesota, experimented with ways to oxygenate blood. By using a simple pump and some tubing, he managed to bypass a dog's heart. He did it by attaching a tube to one lobe of the dog's lung and then directing the blood from the tube through a pump and back into the animal.

Walt Lillehei, Lewis's friend and colleague and one of Minnesota's best cardiac surgeons, was interested in Cohen's research and how it might relate to open-heart surgery. Despite the fact that Cohen had a 90 percent success rate with the fifty dogs he experimented on, both he and Lillehei abandoned the idea of the "self-lung" for use in open-heart surgery. Too many complications arose during the research trials; any kink in the tubing caused blood to flood the animal's lung.

Lillehei brought in another surgeon, Herbert E. Warden, to work on the research. The three men were wondering how Cohen's research could be adapted to make it more workable. Warden, whose wife was pregnant at the time, wondered if they could create something like a placenta, the organ that sends life-sustaining blood from a mother to her unborn child. Not finding anything that could act as a placenta, they decided to hook the patient up to an entire second animal. They called the technique cross circulation. It consisted of inserting tubes into one vein and one artery of a healthy animal, doing the same to the patient, and then attaching the tubes to a machine that pumped oxygenated blood into the patient from the healthy animal. Before they could begin their research, however, they needed a pump and some tubing.

Lillehei decided on a pump used in the dairy industry. The Signamotor Model T-65 pumped liquid in different directions much like the heart; it did not produce the tiny bubbles that can block blood flow, and it cost only $500. The clear tubing they found normally connected barroom taps to beer kegs. The beer hose was easy to sterilize and so cheap that a new, clean length could be used every time.

Cross-circulation trials on dogs showed that a surgeon had a good thirty minutes to operate. The experiments were successful, healing most "patient" dogs and not damaging the "donor" dogs. Lillehei was convinced cross circulation was the answer for open-heart surgery on more complicated congenital defects such as VSD. In late 1953, he found his first human candidate for cross-circulation surgery in baby Gregory Glidden.

The First Cross-Circulation Surgeries

Lyman and Frances Glidden knew what it was like to lose a child to congenital heart disease. In 1950, their twelve-year-old daughter, LaDonnah, suddenly began suffering from high fevers and lung infections. After being in the hospital several times, she was finally diagnosed with VSD. Before anything could be done to help her, LaDonnah's heart gave up, and she died on September 14, 1950.

Born on February 24, 1953, Gregory Glidden began life like his sister LaDonnah, as a healthy infant. But six weeks later Gregory developed symptoms similar to the ones LaDonnah had exhibited. The Gliddens refused to let this child be diagnosed too late for help.

When the doctor heard a heart murmur, X rays were ordered. The radiologist saw an enlarged heart and concluded that Gregory suffered from a hole in his heart—either an ASD or VSD.

The Gliddens were ready to take a chance on Lillehei's experimental surgery to save their son's life. Before the operation could be done, Gregory had to be free of infection. Lillehei ordered antibiotics to clear up the baby's bronchitis.

Though painfully thin and sick, Gregory was a beautiful baby and on most days a happy one. The University of Minnesota hospital staff fell in love with him. "He is cheerful and happy and kicks and plays with his toes in his crib," reported one nurse. "Laughing and waving hands about. Has been playing and cooing most of the evening,"[14] recorded another. It was at the hospital that Gregory said his first word—"Mama"—to a nurse, took his first steps, and celebrated his first birthday. His parents lived a couple of hours away in Hibbing, Minnesota; his father worked as an iron miner, and his mother tended to their other nine children.

On the morning of March 26, 1954, Lillehei performed his first open-heart surgery using cross circulation on Gregory Glidden. Lyman Glidden, Gregory's father, acted as the donor. At 8:30 Gregory was anesthetized with cyclopropane; his chest was opened and his heart exposed. At 8:45 his father was brought in and also anesthetized. Lillehei's assistants cut into Lyman Glidden's right groin to expose the femoral artery, which would carry freshly oxygenated blood to Gregory, and the saphenous vein, which would return the child's oxygen-depleted blood to Lyman's heart. Both Gregory and his father were hooked up to the T-65 milk pump.

At 10:03 the pump was turned on. Gregory's heart was opened but continued to beat. Lillehei quickly found a VSD and sewed it shut. Gregory's heart had been open for ten minutes (much longer than

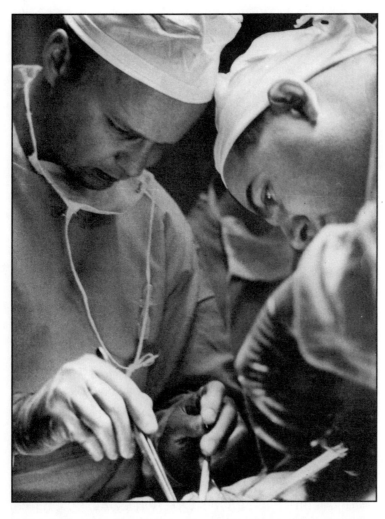

Walt Lillehei performs open-heart surgery on Gregory Glidden on March 26, 1954.

hypothermia would have allowed) when Lillehei began to close it. Lillehei covered the baby's heart with his hand—the murmur and irregular rhythm were both gone; it beat normally. The pump was shut off, Gregory's chest was closed and Lyman Glidden disconnected from it, the incisions in his vessels and groin sewn up. As Lyman awoke, he asked about his son. He was told Gregory was fine.

And Gregory seemed fine. Almost immediately he was eating and sleeping well; rosy color had returned to his cheeks. But a few days later Gregory's condition began to change. At times his lips turned blue, and he

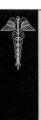

The Queen of Hearts and First Celebrity Patient

In 1954, surgeon Walt Lillehei hosted a press conference. The star of the day was a four-year-old girl with rosy cheeks, big brown eyes, and dark bangs, wearing a ruffly yellow dress. Pamela Schmidt became an instant media darling. A hole in her heart had been surgically closed, and she was well. Her father, Ronald, factory maintenance worker, spoke of her pluck and courage through the ordeal. "She's a fighter," he told reporters at that April 30 conference.

In the next few years, the Minneapolis newspapers did so many stories on the little girl that she became the best-known child in Minnesota in the 1950s. Pictures were published of Pamela riding her bike, playing in the snow, watching herself being interviewed on television, and listening to her mother read her *Squiffy the Skunk*.

She was declared Queen of Hearts, first for the Minnesota Heart Association and then for the American Heart Association. She reigned for several years as a symbol of hope to children suffering from congenital heart defects.

tugged at his ear. His personality also began to change. He cried when held, and he seemed less alert.

On April 2, a nurse reported that Gregory had developed "definite asthmatic type wheezing."[15] On the morning of April 6, 1954, Gregory Glidden was pronounced dead. An autopsy revealed Gregory's heart had healed; pneumonia had killed him.

Lillehei had more success with his next two cross-circulation patients, three-year-old Bradley Mehrman and four-year-old Pamela Schmidt. Like Gregory, their parents acted as their donors. When Lillehei operated on Pamela, the media became interested in this new open-heart procedure. Pamela soon became a celebrity. She appeared on network television and was named the national Queen of Hearts for the American Heart Association.

The Risk Ruins a Life

Though hailed as one of the fathers of open-heart surgery, Lillehei was also accused of taking unnecessary
risks with people's lives by using cross circulation.
One serious failure gave credence to his critics and
damaged his reputation.

On October 5, 1954, Geraldine Thompson, a cross-
circulation donor patient, went into a coma during an
operation to save her daughter Leslie's life. Apparently,
air bubbles had gotten into Geraldine's bloodstream.
She eventually emerged from the coma but was
handicapped and unable to care for herself and her
family.

Lillehei encouraged Geraldine's husband to sue,
telling him, "You can't say I told you that, but the
money you're going to need to take care of Geraldine
for the rest of her life is so great that you won't be
able to handle it on your own."[16] Dan Thompson sued
Lillehei and his assistants for $550,000. The University
of Minnesota Hospital offered to settle the case for
$35,000 and a promise to operate on Leslie for free,
this time using a well-tested heart-lung machine.
Thompson's lawyer convinced Dan to refuse to settle
for less than $50,000. Thompson lost the case and
received nothing for the care of his disabled wife.

After the Thompson operation, Lillehei decided to
use dogs as cross-circulation donor patients. Then, after
finding a better way to perform open-heart surgery,
Lillehei gave up on cross circulation altogether.
Working with a young local doctor, he helped develop
a simple, inexpensive, and effective heart-lung machine.

The First Heart-Lung Machine

Lillehei was the first to develop a relatively small,
efficient heart-lung machine that could be put to frequent use. But he was not the first to build a heart-
lung machine nor the first to use one during
open-heart surgery.

John H. Gibbon Jr. developed the first heart-lung machine over a period of several years. He began working on his machine in the 1930s while training for surgery at Harvard and continued working on it after he became a professor of surgery at Jefferson Medical College in Philadelphia.

Many have described the Gibbon heart-lung machine as big and boxy, like early computers. Its appearance was no accident—Thomas J. Watson, the chairman of IBM, one of the companies that developed the computer, funded Gibbon's work and provided him with technical support.

Searching for a Cross-Circulation Donor

Calvin Richmond was a thirteen-year-old African American from rural Arkansas who had a heart problem. In August of 1954, he fell off a horse-drawn ice truck and was run over by it. Later, doctors at the University of Arkansas determined Calvin had developed a ventricular septal defect (VSD) as a result of the accident. The Arkansas doctors could do nothing for Calvin, but they knew of a doctor in Minnesota who could.

Minnesota was a long way away from Arkansas. Calvin's family had no money to send him there, so the boy became a cause of a Little Rock television station and a local newspaper. School children donated their pennies, the Arkansas Air National Guard offered a plane and pilot to take Calvin to Minnesota, and before long almost $3,000 was collected for the trip and the operation.

Problems arose in Minnesota. Walt Lillehei had agreed to perform his cross-circulation open-heart surgery on Calvin, but he could not find a donor patient. Calvin's mother had refused even without knowing that another mother, Geraldine Thompson, had gone into a coma in a similar situation. Lillehei went to the nearby prison where he had found donor patients in the past. But no prisoner (all were white inmates) would agree to having his blood mingle with that of a black teenager. Finally, Lillehei decided to sedate a large dog, kill it, and harvest its lungs. A beer hose connected the dog's lungs to Calvin, and the old T-65 pump moved freshly oxygenated blood through the boy's body. In twenty minutes Calvin's VSD was repaired.

The day after the operation Calvin spoke to a nurse. Wayne Miller wrote about their conversation in his biography of Walt Lillehei, *King of Hearts*. Calvin asked the nurse why she was taking his blood pressure. "To see if you're alive," she answered. "I'm still talking, ain't I?" he responded. A month later, Calvin left Minnesota, healthy.

Despite the fact that Gibbon never sought out publicity, his machine received a lot of media attention. In 1950, *Life* magazine described Gibbon's creation as "this robot, a gleaming, stainless steel cabinet as big as a piano."[17] The article went on to say that the machine that had successfully substituted for the living heart and lungs of nine dogs for as long as forty-six minutes would soon be tested on human beings. "Soon" was two years later, in 1952, when Gibbon performed open-heart surgery on a fifteen-month-old girl.

Gibbon thought the child had a simple ASD, but the surgery revealed a more complicated problem. The toddler died on the operating table. A year later Gibbon was successful when he operated on eighteen-year-old Cecelia Bavolek, repairing her simple ASD. Bavolek went home from the hospital after only thirteen days, cured. Gibbon was not so fortunate with several operations that followed. He became discouraged and gave up open-heart surgery for a year.

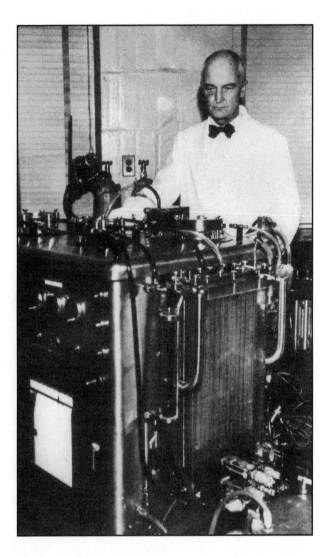

John H. Gibbon Jr. stands beside his heart-lung machine.

In 1945, Clarence Dennis, a surgeon at the University of Minnesota Hospital, visited Gibbon in Philadelphia. Dennis wanted to learn more about Gibbon's machine, and he received permission to take Gibbon's blueprints back with him to Minneapolis.

There Dennis worked for years modifying Gibbon's design. After experimenting with his version of a heart-lung machine, Dennis became the first to use such a device in open-heart surgery on a human being. On April 6, 1951, Dennis tested his modified machine on six-year-old Patty Anderson. The heart-lung machine worked, but it was so complicated that four people were needed to operate it. Unfortunately, Patty's heart had deteriorated to a point where surgery could not save her, and she died.

Walt Lillehei watched Dennis operate. Fascinated by Patty's surgery, Lillehei was inspired to find a way to make heart-lung machines more effective.

The Minnesota Machines

Dr. Richard DeWall was bored with practicing medicine, but he liked to tinker in his spare time. Wanting to use his skills and interests to develop medical technology and conduct research, he approached Walt Lillehei about a job. All Lillehei had to offer DeWall was a part-time job at the university hospital's animal research lab. Still, the young doctor jumped at the chance. DeWall worked hard, and before long he was promoted to pump technician.

In 1955, Lillehei asked DeWall to help build an oxygenator for open-heart surgery. Lillehei stressed that "it had to be something simple."[18]

DeWall began experimenting with laboratory dogs. He soon discovered blood with bubbles was lighter than blood without bubbles. Bubbling blood rose to the top of any container. He further realized that it was much easier for smaller bubbles to slip into the bloodstream, putting a patient in danger. DeWall used this knowledge to build a machine that cost less than $15 to make and had no moving parts other than the T-65 pump Lillehei used in cross-circulation procedures. It worked by feeding oxygen-depleted blood into a plastic tube, where large bubbles of oxygen were introduced through eighteen needles. Carbon dioxide was released as the blood absorbed oxygen, just like in a human lung. Then the oxygenated blood flowed past an antifoaming agent (a product used in the dairy industry) and down through a beer hose as the remaining bubbles rose to the top of the stream and burst. The pump then returned the bubble-free oxygenated blood to the patient. DeWall and Lillehei ran several successful tests of the machine on laboratory dogs before using it for open-heart surgery on human patients.

Two hours away from the University of Minnesota Hospital, John W. Kirklin was working on his own

The DeWall heart-lung machine undergoes its first test on July 12, 1955.

heart-lung machine at the Mayo Clinic in Rochester, Minnesota. Kirklin tried to improve on Gibbon's machine. What he built cost a thousand times more than the DeWall-Lillehei heart-lung machine. It was as large as a piano and required a technician to operate it. But by 1955, it was working well, and Kirklin was using it with patients needing open-heart surgery.

The state of Minnesota could boast of having the only two surgeons in the country who regularly performed open-heart surgery. But they were not the only surgeons interested in operating on open hearts.

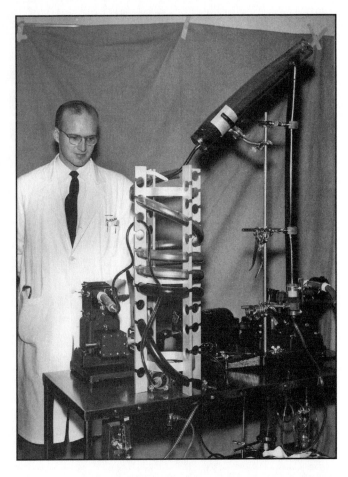

The Cooley Coffee Pot

In 1954 at a meeting of the Southern Surgical Society in Hot Springs, Virginia, Denton Cooley expressed his interest in developing a new heart-lung machine. Cooley wanted his hospital, St. Luke's in Houston, Texas, to enter the open-heart surgery field.

Cooley considered improving upon what Gibbon had designed, but then he decided to build his own heart-lung machine. C. J. Tibideau, a Houston oil broker and Cooley's close friend, gave the surgeon $5,000 to finance the project. Cooley found most of his machine's materials at the local hardware store. What he could not find there, he had made in metal shops. A commercial kitchen supply company produced the major custom work, and for that reason the Cooley heart-lung machine was referred to as the "Cooley Coffee Pot." Its official name was the Mark-Cooley heart-lung machine.

The first laboratory trials killed a lot of dogs, but Cooley was not discouraged. He rationalized: "Anyone who had worked in an animal lab knows how easily an animal dies, particularly dogs. They're fragile. They are not endowed with a constitution or a will to live and, consequently, are poor human substitutes."[19]

Cooley got a call from Dr. Sidney Schnur about a patient who had developed multiple VSDs as a result of a heart attack. Without further testing on laboratory dogs, Cooley decided to use his heart-lung machine on a human patient. "We put Mr. Sommerville on the pump and I patched up the holes in his ventricular septum. He survived for six weeks before dying of an infection, but that was time enough to get us on the road,"[20] said Cooley. Before Sommerville died, Cooley did six more, less difficult, open-heart surgeries.

Cooley ordered two more heart-lung machines built, and he began performing open-heart surgery on a regular basis.

With the development and refinement of the heart-lung machine, more and more surgeons ventured into the field of open-heart surgery. Now that surgeons had the time to deal with complicated conditions, they began to develop techniques to replace damaged parts of the heart. Eventually, some even wondered about replacing diseased hearts with healthy ones.

CHAPTER 3

The First Transplant

"The time is ripe for a human heart transplant," cardiac researcher Norm Shumway was quoted as saying in a 1967 issue of a medical journal. "The required conditions being that a recipient and a compatible donor turn up simultaneously."21

Whether or not they read Shumway's interview, many cardiac surgeons believed it to be true, and some even dreamed of being the first to perform a human heart transplant. After all, a lot was at stake: the chance to make medical history while prolonging a life that would otherwise be lost to heart disease, the development of a cutting-edge medical program at their hospitals, and a chance to gain international renown.

Much had happened in the field of cardiac surgery between the mid-1950s and 1967. New developments had turned once complex operations into routine procedures, saving countless lives. Open-heart surgery programs had been introduced in medical centers throughout the United States and the world, spawned by a new kind of surgeon, ambitious and politically aware. The old leaders in the field lost some status. University of Minnesota chief surgeon Owen Wangensteen retired, and Walt Lillehei moved on to New York. But other heart surgery innovations were to emerge.

Lone Star State Legends

To most Americans in the 1960s, the pioneers in open-heart surgery were two doctors from Houston, Texas. Michael DeBakey performed heart surgery like it was an art form—beautifully. Denton Cooley was known for the speed and precision with which he worked. "Denton operates so fast," Dwight Harken once said, "that he could get away with anything!"[22]

Each recognized the value of publicizing his work. DeBakey believed strongly in self-promotion. "He is a master of publicity. He was the first doctor to realize what a valuable tool it could be,"[23] said one DeBakey watcher. DeBakey was also a prolific writer in medical journals, a doctor's primary source of information for new medical developments.

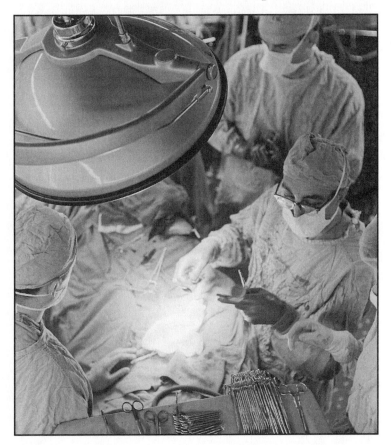

Dr. Michael DeBakey performs cardiovascular surgery at Houston's Methodist Hospital on December 12, 1964.

Both men had loyal followers as well as critics. One scrub nurse who worked with Cooley declared, "I've had it with Dr. Wonderful and his God Squad. I'll take orthopedics!"[24]

Together, they made Houston a launching pad for the new frontier of cardiac surgery. In 1948, DeBakey was hired to upgrade the department of surgery at Baylor College of Medicine in Houston. DeBakey accomplished the task through the willing support and funding of the city of Houston. In 1952, he hired Cooley, and within a decade the two built up Houston's reputation as a heart surgery center while further bringing cardiac surgery in general into the limelight.

DeBakey and Cooley did more heart operations than any other surgeons anywhere. The sheer volume of operations performed by DeBakey and Cooley became legendary. Once DeBakey performed eleven elaborate operations in the span of eighteen and one-half hours. When he was through at 1:30 A.M., he stuck his head out into the empty hospital corridor and asked, "Anybody else out there want an operation?"[25]

Visiting surgeons could observe more heart surgeries in Houston in a week than elsewhere in months. As a result of the volume of surgeries performed, patients from all over the world flocked to the Texas city in hopes of being helped by DeBakey and Cooley.

By 1955, heart-lung machines were convenient and efficient, allowing surgeons to pursue more complex operations. Cardiac surgery research propelled by men like Michael DeBakey and Denton Cooley continued at an even quicker pace in the 1960s, laying the groundwork for human heart transplantation and the development of the artificial heart.

Latest Developments Become Routine

Surgeons first looked to replacing defective heart parts. Artificial valves that could replace diseased ones were developed and successfully implanted into patients. Charles Hufnagel, a Boston surgeon, installed the first caged-ball type artificial valve in the thoracic aorta in 1952. Dwight Harken surgically replaced an aortic valve with an artificial one in 1960, and Albert Starr, a Portland, Oregon, surgeon, replaced a patient's mitral valve with an artificial one in 1961.

While valve replacement saved many lives, two other operations became even more widely used. One is the installation of a pacemaker, a surgically implanted device that sends electrical pulses to the heart, helping it maintain a normal rhythm. Rapid or uneven heartbeats can kill patients if not corrected. In 1952 Paul Zoll, a Boston surgeon, developed an external pacemaker, and in 1959 Swiss surgeon Ake Senning installed the first totally implanted pacemaker in a patient.

Heart Shock

The scene of Dr. Frankenstein with the "creature" strapped to a gurney while lightning strikes is the stuff of fiction. Yet the life-giving and life-endangering characteristics of electricity have fascinated mankind since ancient times. Records indicate one of Roman emperor Nero's slaves was saved from death by the shock of an electric eel. In the nineteenth century, Italian scientists tried to revive cadavers with electrical current, and German researchers discovered that applying electricity to the bodies of recently beheaded criminals made their hearts beat.

Much later, electrical shock was succesfully used to restart and restore natural rhythm to a still heart. In 1947, Cleveland surgeon Claude Beck developed the first defibrillator, which applied a strong electrical shock to the heart to correct an irregular heartbeat. Defibrillators are emergency room staples today because they counteract cardiac arrest. Pacemakers help maintain normal heartbeats. Both pacemakers and defibrillators developed from similar research on electrical shock and the heart.

The first pacemaker, developed in the 1930s, was not implanted in the patient but used like a probe that was inserted into the chest cavity to electrically stimulate the heart. Albert Hyman, a New York City doctor, is credited with designing this early device. Unlike the media-savvy heart surgeons of the 1960s, Hyman did not promote his creation. It would take a few more decades before Hyman's invention would be appreciated.

In 1957, Lillehei worked with a television repairman named Earl Bakken to design a semi-implantable and portable pacemaker that was powered by a regular nine-volt battery. Bakken would go on to design an implantable pacemaker, as would Paul Zoll, who developed the first widely used external pacemaker.

Today's pacemakers ensure that a heart keeps beating normally whether the patient is physically active or at rest. Boston surgeon Dwight Harken called the modern pacemaker operation "a very simple affair now done under local anesthetic."[26] By 1978, nearly three hundred thousand pacemakers had been manufactured and implanted in patients.

The other operation is the coronary artery bypass, in which a length of vein is used to redirect the flow of blood from a blocked artery to the heart. The coronary bypass was developed by Rene Favaloro of Cleveland, Ohio, in 1967. Twelve years later, in 1978, more than seventy-five thousand bypass operations had been performed, eleven thousand of those by one surgeon, Denton Cooley of Houston.

Heart valve repair, pacemakers, and bypass surgery saved many lives and provided heart surgeons with a

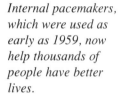

Internal pacemakers, which were used as early as 1959, now help thousands of people have better lives.

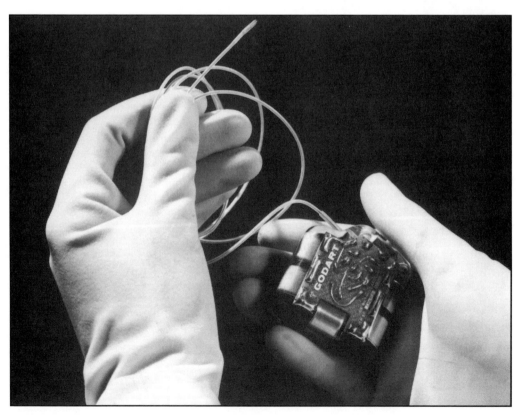

wealth of experience. When such procedures became commonplace, many high-profile surgeons looked for further breakthroughs—they wanted to be the first to perform a human heart transplant. "I was eager to participate," said Cooley. "I discussed the matter with my associates. I told them I was contemplating doing a transplant and to be on the lookout for a donor."[27]

However, Cooley would not be the first surgeon to perform a human heart transplant, nor would he develop the procedures for such a complex operation. Other surgeons and researchers would be involved in that historic surgery.

Early Transplant Attempts Inform Doctors About Rejection

The first heart transplant and heart-lung transplant experiments took place in the early twentieth century. In 1905, Alexis Carrel and Charles Guthrie at the University of Chicago transplanted the heart of a small dog into the neck of a larger dog. The larger dog's new heart beat at a rate of eighty-eight times per minute. (Normal heart rate for dogs is one hundred beats per minute.) The dog survived only a few hours after the surgery. Shortly thereafter, Carrel and Guthrie unsuccessfully attempted to transplant the heart and lungs of a week-old kitten into the neck of an adult cat.

In 1922, Frank Mann at the Mayo Clinic in Rochester, Minnesota, tried transplant experiments similar to those done by Carrel and Guthrie and had similar results. While Carrel, Guthrie, and Mann did not develop a method of heart transplantation, they learned an important fact from their studies. "It is readily seen that the failure of the transplanted heart to survive is not due to the technique of transplantation," wrote Mann, "but to some biological factor which is probably identical to that which prevents survival of other homotransplanted tissues and organs."[28] In other words, those early researchers realized rejection

Animal Hearts and Human Patients

In the mid-1960s, many cardiac surgeons sought patients and donors for the first human heart transplant. Early in 1964 James Hardy had found both. Like Norman Shumway and Richard Lower at Stanford, Hardy and his team at the University of Mississippi had done hundreds of experimental heart transplants with animals. Following Shumway's method, they worked mostly with young calves instead of dogs.

Hardy learned of an elderly man with a long-standing heart condition whose leg had been amputated. The surgeon was determined to save the man's life. In a nearby ward was a young man with irreversible brain damage. The young man's family agreed to donate his heart for the first transplant once they were sure he could not live any longer.

Unfortunately, the condition of the elderly man did not allow Hardy to wait for the human donor, but the hearts of university lab animals were available. Two large chimpanzees were brought as possible donors. Hardy and his team decided to go ahead with a chimpanzee heart in what would be the first animal-to-human organ transplant. The operation was considered a temporary measure until a human donor became available.

The elderly man's heart gave out with the first incision, but his blood continued to circulate through a heart-lung machine. Hardy removed the human heart and replaced it with the chimp's heart. One electric shock and the borrowed animal heart began to beat, but it was too small to handle the demands of the human body. To compensate, surgeons made the transplanted heart beat faster. It worked for a short time, but three hours later the chimp heart failed even before antirejection drugs could be administered.

of foreign organs would be a serious problem in any transplant attempt.

Years later, in 1940, Russian surgeon Vladimir Demikhov also tried heart transplantation in animals. His research was interrupted by World War II. When he resumed his study in 1946, he was the first researcher to transplant a dog's heart into the organ's normal location in another dog. Some of his animals lived for a few days, but Demikhov became discouraged, ultimately believing such a surgery was too complex.

In 1953, Wilford Neptune and Charles Bailey at Hahnemann University in Philadelphia conducted another series of animal heart transplant experiments. They used previous transplant techniques and hypothermia (reducing the animal's temperature), with results no better than Demikhov's.

Then in the late 1950s, a former intern at the University of Minnesota who had gone on to be a Stanford University surgeon, began experiments that eventually led to the procedure for human heart transplantation.

The Shumway Technique

In the old pair of sneakers and rumpled green medical smock he usually wore, Norman Shumway did not look or act like a pioneering heart surgeon. Shumway studied the effects of hypothermia with F. John Lewis at the University of Minnesota in the 1950s. There he was fondly known for his irreverent behavior and wry sense of humor. Chief surgeon Owen Wangensteen was annoyed when one of his patients kept mistaking him for Walt Lillehei. The woman kept insisting Wangensteen was not who he was when he visited her. Shumway went up to the chief surgeon, put his arm around him, and said, "You've got to stop this going around the hospital telling everyone you're Dr. Wangensteen."[29]

Serious about his studies, Shumway continued his research on hypothermia when he moved on to Stanford University in California. Specifically, Shumway studied what is called the ventricular fibrillation threshold. In ventricular fibrillation, the ventricles function irregularly so that the

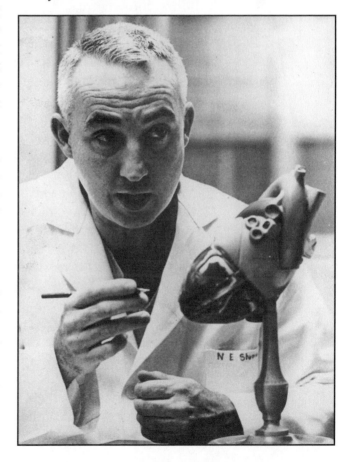

Dr. Norman Shumway, renowned for his work in heart transplantation, discusses a model of the human heart.

heart cannot pump. A defibrillator—a device that uses electrical shock—can often return a heart to normal rhythm. Shumway found that as the temperature of the heart fell, less electrical current was needed to defibrillate, or start the heart beating normally again.

Shumway and fellow researcher Richard Lower got bored while waiting for research animal hearts to cool down. "All sorts of fantasies were indulged in while waiting,"[30] wrote Shumway. To pass the time, the two surgically removed dog hearts and then reattached them—a method referred to as autotransplantation. Then in December 1959, Shumway and Lower successfully performed an animal heart transplant. In contrast to similar earlier efforts, many of the dogs in Shumway's and Lower's experiments lived for weeks, instead of days or hours, and were active, with a normal tolerance for exercise, before they died. Lower referred to their first transplant as a "technical stunt"[31] because he realized there were still significant problems to overcome—such as the body's rejecting the organ—before heart transplantation could become a reality.

Shumway and Lower did discover one way to help fight rejection. Rejection happens when the body's immune system recognizes foreign tissue—such as a donor heart—and defends the body against it much like it would fight disease-causing organisms like bacteria or viruses. Medications that suppress the immune system help the body cope with a transplanted organ, but they also make the body more susceptible to infection. Shumway and Lower found that slowing the heart's functions with hypothermia and using less voltage to restore heart function minimized the side effects of these immunosuppressive medications and helped prevent infection. Although the problem of transplant rejection still seemed overwhelming, Shumway was encouraged. In 1960, he said that if a better way of dealing with rejection were developed, the transplanted hearts of his laboratory dogs "would continue to function adequately for the normal life span of the animal."[32]

Within a few years, the development of drugs that fight the body's resistance to foreign tissue brought the prospect of human heart transplantation closer to reality. That first successful human-to-human heart transplant was not performed by Shumway at Stanford, by Cooley in Texas, or by Lillehei in Minnesota. It was performed by a relatively unknown surgeon in Cape Town, South Africa.

Holding on to Make History

"I know it's a phrase that's been used a lot these days, but when you see it happen, when you see a man struggling along with a heart two-thirds dead, you can only say you've seen something really remarkable about a human being,"[33] said Barry Kaplan, a Cape Town, South Africa, doctor about his patient Louis Washkansky.

By all accounts, fifty-three-year-old Washkansky was a courageous man. But one of the most courageous things he ever did was to stay alive long enough to make medical history. In April 1966 Washkansky and his wife, Ann, came to see Kaplan because neither of them could sleep at night. Louis had trouble breathing; he was so short of breath that it scared his wife. "I know as soon as I close my eyes," Ann told the doctor, "that he will take a real long one [breath] and never breathe anymore."[34]

Washkansky had been diagnosed with heart trouble before, but he assumed his current problem had to do with his lungs. Kaplan soon found that Washkansky suffered from Cheyne-Stokes breathing, and it was caused by gross heart failure. "It's rather terrifying to witness," said Kaplan of Cheyne-Stokes. "The patient takes a short breath then a deeper one, then a still deeper one—going on like that until he stops breathing altogether, lying there with no sign of respiration."[35]

This was the most serious condition in a long line of illnesses that Louis Washkansky had endured. In

1950, he suffered his first heart attack; in 1955, he was diagnosed with diabetes; in 1960, he suffered another heart attack and another in 1965. All of those events had severely weakened his heart.

Washkansky was not a man to complain—ever. Even when he was at his worst and his wife asked him how he was, he would say, "I'm on top of the world." But in 1967, it became more difficult for Washkansky to deny or ignore his health problems. An X ray of his heart revealed it to be huge. Kaplan described it as the biggest heart he had ever seen, only one inch from the left border of Louis's chest and only two inches from the right. "I gave him a very bad prognosis, certainly no more than a couple of months," wrote Kaplan. "Yet this man struggled on for two and a half years before the operation."[36]

On the morning of December 3, 1967, Louis Washkansky asked his cardiac surgeon, "Aren't you going to give me a new heart?"

"Yes," the surgeon answered. "So it's out with the old and in with the new. . . . Auld Lang Syne."[37]

Perhaps the most courageous thing Louis Washkansky ever did was to put his faith and his life in the hands of a South African surgeon by the name of Christiaan Barnard.

The First Human Heart Transplant

Forty-five-year-old Christiaan Barnard was handsome, charming, and ambitious. Barnard had trained at the University of Minnesota under Walt Lillehei. In early 1967, Barnard spent three months at the Medical College of Virginia gaining clinical experience in kidney transplantation. There he observed Richard Lower doing a heart transplant on a dog.

After returning to his native South Africa, Barnard helped start a kidney transplant program at Groote Schuur Hospital in Cape Town. The one and only kidney transplant he performed was a success, and he was anxious to do more cardiac surgery. Specifically, he felt ready to attempt a human-to-human heart transplant.

Barnard badgered the head of the hospital cardiac unit, Dr. Velva Schrire, to help him find a suitable candidate for a transplant. Barnard and Schrire both agreed that the patient should have irreversible heart disease, should have failed to benefit from other forms of treatment, and be close to death. In the first week of November 1967, Schrire found a patient who fit those criteria: Louis Washkansky.

Washkansky agreed to the operation, so it was a matter of finding the right donor heart. Schrire and Barnard would only accept donors whose medical histories showed that they were without heart disease, under age thirty-five, and did not suffer from diabetes or

Apartheid and Heart Transplants

Until 1990, black and white South Africans lived separately under a strict policy of racial segregation known as apartheid. The white minority, of Dutch descent and known as Afrikaners, had control of the government. Nonwhite South Africans, including those of mixed race, were discriminated against in housing, employment, and public services. South Africa had long been criticized for apartheid. Christiaan Barnard was sensitive to world opinion and to those struggling under apartheid.

Barnard admitted Louis Washkansky's heart transplant could have occurred two weeks earlier when a suitable black donor was found. Years later, Barnard wrote about his concerns in *History of Transplantation: Thirty-Five Recollections*: "Professor Schrire and I decided that the first patient and donor for heart transplantation should be white South Africans, not because of any problems with South African authorities but because we were afraid that if either the patient or donors were black we would be criticized for having experimented on black patients."

After that first operation, things changed. Twenty-four-year-old Clive Haupt was of mixed race—known in South Africa as one of the Cape Coloreds. On New Year's Day, 1968, Clive collapsed while on a picnic with his wife Dorothy. Doctors determined he had a massive cerebral hemorrhage. At the hospital, Dorothy and Clive's mother, who worked as a cleaning lady, gave their permission for Clive's heart to be used for Barnard's second heart transplant operation. "If you can save the life of another person, take my son's heart," Clive's mother was quoted as saying in Barnard's first memoir. Barnard's patient, Philip Blaiberg, agreed to accept Haupt's heart, in fact, any heart. Perhaps, because like Louis Washkansky, Philip Blaiberg was the son of Jewish immigrants, he did not share the racial prejudice felt by most Dutch-descended white Afrikaners.

hypertension. One was found on December 2, 1967. "It was Saturday afternoon and I was having a nap when Dr. Bosman phoned to tell me that he thought we had a donor,"[38] wrote Barnard. The donor was Denise Davall, a twenty-four-year-old woman who was pronounced brain-dead after suffering injuries from an automobile accident near the hospital.

In the early hours of December 3, 1967, Louis Washkansky was prepped for surgery. When Louis was about to be anesthetized, the nurse asked if he would lie down. "Can't you do it while I'm sitting up?" asked Washkansky. "No," she replied. Dr. Ozinsky, the anesthesiologist, added "You have to recline. These surgeons are worse than movie stars. They don't like anyone stealing their limelight."[39] Barnard credited Ozinsky's sense of humor with helping Washkansky relax before surgery.

At 2:32 A.M. the donor heart went into arrest— that is, it stopped beating. Only then could it be

Dr. Christiaan Barnard's medical team works on a patient in the same room where the Washkansky heart transplant took place just days earlier.

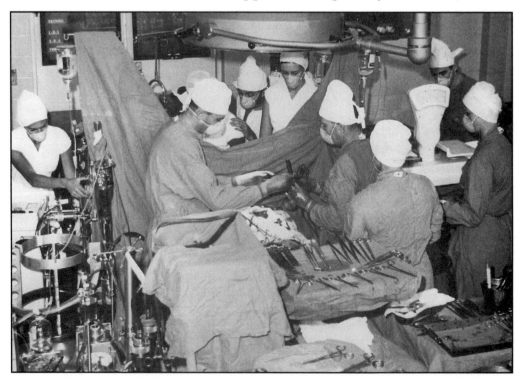

removed from Denise Davall's body and connected to an oxygenator. At the same time, Louis Washkansky was hooked up to a heart-lung machine, the DeWall-Lillehei bubble oxygenator, and his body was cooled.

At 3:01 A.M. Barnard removed Louis Washkansky's heart. "This was a heart for history," Barnard later wrote. "Equal to the man who carried it, the man who refused to lie down and give up. And now, there was little left—other than to watch it die. The fibrillation, tragic spasms heralding the end, became more aggravated. The heart which God had given to Louis Washkansky was approaching its moment of death."[40]

Attaching the donor heart was a fairly simple procedure. Following the Shumway technique, Barnard joined the left atria, or upper chamber, of the donor heart to the recipient first; then the right atria was joined; then the pulmonary arteries and the aorta were sutured into place.

At 5:43 A.M. the first human-to-human heart transplant was completed. By 8:30 A.M. anesthesia was discontinued, and Louis was returned to a special ward and placed on a ventilator. Barnard left the hospital soon afterward. There was no crowd of reporters waiting for him, but on his way home Barnard did hear a news bulletin about the operation on his car radio.

At 9 A.M. on December 4, 1967, Washkansky was taken off the ventilator and placed in an oxygen tent. Louis was now able to talk for the first time since his surgery. Barnard asked him if he knew what had happened. Louis answered: "You promised me a new heart. . . . I assume you kept your promise."[41] Louis began taking medications to help ensure that his body would not reject the heart.

Washkansky lived for eighteen days after the transplant. The autopsy showed a blue and dead heart perfectly sutured into place; it was pneumonia that had killed Louis Washkansky.

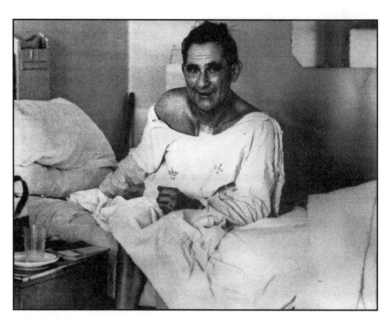

Louis Washkansky sits up in his hospital bed after undergoing cardiac transplant surgery.

Louis Washkansky will forever be known as a brave man willing to risk his life to save it. Between surgeon and patient, Barnard and Washkansky changed cardiac surgery and the way the heart is thought of forever.

The Immediate Aftermath

Barnard was hailed as both a saint and a sinner; his accomplishment was the biggest news story of its day. Barnard became an instant hero in his native South Africa. He appeared on television talk shows and received high praise from renowned colleagues. Walt Lillehei called Barnard's operation a "fantastic piece of surgery." In Houston, Michael DeBakey called it "a real breakthrough!"[42] Denton Cooley sent his congratulations to Barnard on his first heart transplant in a cablegram, adding, "I will be reporting on my first hundred soon."[43]

Even though several surgeons had been preparing to perform heart transplants, the news of Barnard's feat came as a surprise to the world medical community. "Like most surgeons, I was dumbfounded when I heard that Chris Barnard had done a transplant, and I immediately predicted failure within forty-eight hours," wrote Denton Cooley. "The truth is, I was envious of Barnard. I wished very much it had been me."[44]

Perhaps the most interesting reaction to this medical milestone was the intensified competition to be the next to perform a human heart transplant. Three days after Barnard's operation, New York surgeon Adrian

Blaiberg in the Spotlight

When Dr. Christiaan Barnard first saw fifty-eight-year-old Philip Blaiberg, he was reminded of a Christmas icon. "He looked like Santa Claus, with a tubby belly, red cheeks, blue eyes and a big mouth—except this was no laughing Santa," said Barnard. "His mouth was open and [he was] gasping for air." This Cape Town dentist was about to become almost as famous as Santa. He was the second man to receive a new heart in an operation performed by Barnard.

Blaiberg kept his old heart preserved in a jar, and he had no qualms about showing it to visitors or the rash of reporters waiting to interview him. To Blaiberg that old heart was a symbol of how well he was, and he was only too happy to share that news with the rest of the world—a world that was fascinated by his ordeal.

When Blaiberg left Groote Schuur Hospital in March 1968, he insisted on leaving his wheelchair at the exit door and walking to his car unassisted. A crowd of photographers clicked away as he went to the waiting car. He also walked by himself from the car to the front door of his Cape Town apartment. Only when he was out of sight of the press did he ask for help—help which he really needed. But when anyone doubted the extent of his recovery, he challenged them to come see for themselves.

Blaiberg lived for an impressive 551 days—almost all of them in the spotlight. He tried to hide it, but Blaiberg was far less healthy than he allowed the world to see. Throughout those 551 days, he suffered several setbacks, often becoming dangerously ill. On August 17, 1969, his borrowed heart finally gave out completely.

Philip Blaiberg leaves Groote Schuur Hospital on March 16, 1968.

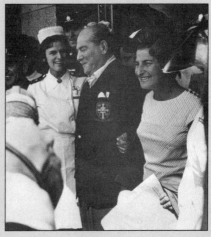

Kantrowitz replaced the heart of a two-week-old infant with the heart from a baby born without a brain. The recipient lived only a few hours. On January 2, 1968, Barnard performed his second heart transplant. The donor heart came from a man of mixed race named Clive Haupt; the recipient was a white South African named Philip Blaiberg. (South Africa was racially segregated at that time.) Blaiberg survived a remarkable 551 days after the operation and became the most famous patient in the world.

Countless surgeons joined the race, including Shumway, who transplanted a heart from a brain-dead woman into a fifty-four-year-old man on Januanry 6, 1968. Universities and hospitals all over the world set up heart transplant programs, performing 101 heart transplants in 1968 alone.

Cooley finally performed his first heart transplant in May of that same year. By that time it seemed to many that this contest was as much about gratifying surgeons' egos as it was for the good of humanity. While Cooley maintained that his first concern was saving lives, he admitted that "it would be untrue to say that I was not eager to take part in this, the most exciting development in cardiac surgery"[45] and that he was frustrated in not being able to find a donor heart until fairly late in the game.

Amid the frenzy, serious questions and issues arose that would have to be dealt with if human heart transplantation was to remain a viable medical procedure for those at death's door.

CHAPTER 4

Increasing Transplant Life Expectancy

The desire of cardiac surgeons to become skilled at heart transplantation increased throughout 1968 despite mounting evidence that the operation neither promised long-term survival nor a better quality of life to patients. This situation amazed many heart doctors. "There ensued what appeared to be an international race to be a member of the me-too brigade. There has not been anything like it in medical annals,"[46] wrote cardiologist Irvine Page.

It seemed the excitement over the new technique blinded many experienced surgeons to its limitations. "There is no question in my mind that heart transplants can be done with very low risk—say, 5 percent mortality," said Denton Cooley in 1968. "It will become a routine operation during the next decade. . . . It's only a question now of resolving such details as body rejection and getting people to accept the idea of walking around with someone else's heart."[47] As Cooley and others would soon come to learn, tackling the problem of rejection, overturning long-held beliefs about the heart and its function, and finding donor hearts were not details but major obstacles.

63

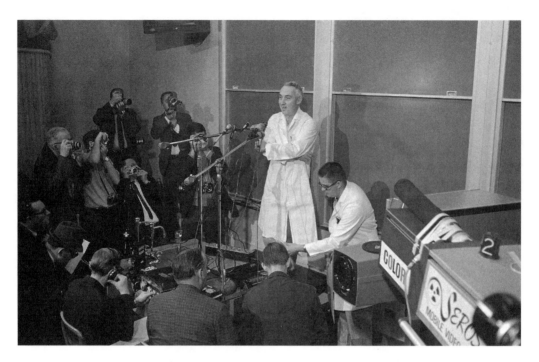

Dr. Norman Shumway speaks at a press conference about the complications of his first heart transplant, which he completed in January 1968.

Euphoria Dies

A few surgeons, such as Boston's Dwight Harken, an early cardiac pioneer, warned of replacing diseased hearts until the problem of rejection could be brought under control. But warnings were not as effective in slowing enthusiasm for heart transplantation as the increasing score of deaths. Of the 101 recipients of donor hearts in 1968, only three lived beyond a year. Philip Blaiberg, Barnard's second transplant, was one, living more than a year and a half after his operation. The other two managed to survive until 1977; one had a transplant in Milwaukee, Wisconsin, and the other in Marseilles, France.

Watching their patients suffer complications and reject "new" hearts took a great toll on cardiac surgeons, who had a difficult enough time dealing with the lives of their patients. Houston surgeon Don Bricker says:

> There's simply no area of surgery where you can lose patients on the table as you do in heart work. Gunshots,

traffic-crushed victims—these patients may crater on you. But with elective [treatment a patient and doctor choose] heart surgery, you're the guy who makes the decision to operate, and when you fix the heart and it doesn't start up again, then you're the guy who killed him. When it happens to me, I go out and sit somewhere and weep.[48]

There was no telling when rejection might reverse the progress made. But rejection was not the only problem heart transplant surgeons faced.

Norman Shumway performed his first heart transplant in January 1968, and the operation was fraught with trouble. The patient, a fifty-four-year-old steelworker named Mike Casparak, was dying from chronic viral myocarditis, an inflammation of the heart. The donor heart came from a forty-three-year-old woman. Casparak's diseased heart had grown so large that the body cavity it sat in was three times the size of the donor heart. The situation caused a multitude of technical problems. After the five-hour operation, the patient required a vast volume of transfused blood. Two days later, Casparak's liver and kidneys failed, and he was bleeding in his stomach. Eventually, Casparak lapsed into a coma and died. The hospital bill for the operation and recovery time was $28,845—almost $2,000 per day for fifteen postoperative days. Many in the medical community objected to the expense, saying the money could have been better used elsewhere.

Of Denton Cooley's first three transplant patients, two died quickly. By August 1968, after having transplanted nine hearts, only six of those patients were still alive. Cooley was criticized for operating on an Alpine, Texas, hospital administrator named James Stuckwish. At a medical meeting, several colleagues told Cooley that Stuckwish was too ill to survive a transplant. Stuckwish had one heart attack just hours before his surgery and another during the operation. Stuckwish survived the transplant operation only to have his kidney and liver shut down, killing him seven days later. Cooley answered his critics sharply:

There are few surgeons in the world who would try what we did on Stuckwish. We don't refuse to operate on patients if they are too sick, only if they're not sick enough. The real issue here is not are we going to offer a transplant to a man, but are we going to deny it to someone who is in the last hour of his life! . . . Stuckwish's case illustrates dramatically that a transplant has real therapeutic clinical value. We have demonstrated that resuscitation of a patient by transplant is possible.[49]

A Heart Revisited

Denton Cooley was looking to do his first heart transplant on forty-seven-year-old Everett Thomas, whose heart had been badly damaged by rheumatic fever. The surgeon gave an account of the operation in Henry Minetree's biography, *Cooley*. "When I learned a potential donor was in the hospital," said Cooley, "I immediately thought of Thomas. He was a comparatively young man, and other than a ruined heart and some paralysis, the rest of his body was in pretty good shape. The young lady, of course, was hopeless. She was decerebrate [brain-dead] and the bullet was lodged in the base of her brain."

As fate would have it, Cooley knew the fifteen-year-old gunshot victim who would become the donor for Thomas's surgery. She was Katherine Martin, and Cooley had operated on her for a coarctation, or a narrowing of the aorta, when she was nine years old. "It was a peculiar coincidence that this girl should arrive as a potential donor," Cooley said. When he operated on Martin, her heart had been enlarged from the stress of a constricted aorta. Cooley said, "But now, as a replacement for the diseased heart of a large man, this cardiac enlargment was so much the better to handle his circulation."

Martin's heart was transplanted into Thomas in the early morning hours of May 4, 1968. The operation took a mere thirty-five minutes, and Thomas went on to live nearly six months more before succumbing to rejection.

Dr. Denton Cooley describes Everett Thomas's heart transplant operation.

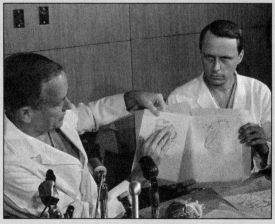

Two Hearts Better than One

In the mid 1970s and early 1980s, Christiaan Barnard had some success with implanting "spare" hearts in patients whose diseased hearts were barely functioning. The operation was not exactly a transplant because the patient's diseased heart was not removed when a donor heart was implanted into the chest cavity. Together the two hearts supported one another and the patient's circulatory system.

In many cases the procedure helped the diseased heart somewhat recover, becoming more functional. Rejection of the implanted heart was not fatal. The donor heart did not have to be as healthy as a donor heart for a regular transplant, which made finding donors easier.

By 1981, Barnard had performed thirty of these surgeries. Sixty percent of his patients survived for more than a year after the operation. A few survived for five years.

Denton Cooley considered doing the "spare" heart procedure for selected high-risk patients but never attempted it. Barnard abandoned the procedure eventually when the development of artificial devices to assist diseased hearts became a reality.

Upon years of reflection, Christiaan Barnard came to disagree with Cooley's view on who should be eligible for heart transplantation. In the 1990s, Barnard wrote that with the first transplants he too believed that no potential patient could be too ill or too old for the operation. "Looking back now," he said, "we recognize that this was a mistake and was the reason for many of the failures in the early days of cardiac transplantation. It was not that patients did not benefit from their new hearts but the terminally ill patient, especially associated with certain complications, did not do well on the high doses of steroids that were used before the introduction of cyclosporine."[50]

The overall results of those first 101 heart transplants in 1968 were so discouraging that only 47 were attempted in 1969. Many surgeons felt a need to step back and examine the problems associated with transplantation before performing more surgery. Denton Cooley was not among that group. "Nonsense," said Cooley to the idea of a moratorium on heart transplantation. "We don't have enough patients done yet to assess the results. Every case that is attempted proves the validity of the concept."[51]

Making the Odds Better with Donor Heart Biopsies

Norman Shumway watched as the method he developed led to near hysteria in support of human heart transplantation. He also saw that hysteria die within a year, to be replaced by a negative view of the surgery by both the medical community and the press. "Both reactions are probably inappropriate," Shumway said. "At this point, we believe cardiac transplantation remains within the realm of clinical investigation."[52] Shumway knew lives were prolonged through heart transplantation, and he was hopeful that new developments would allow patients to survive longer. But like Cooley, Shumway knew that only through more research and more surgery would heart transplantation enter the medical mainstream.

Heart transplant patient Keith Castle poses for photographs with his wife and daughter at his bed at Papworth Hospital in 1970.

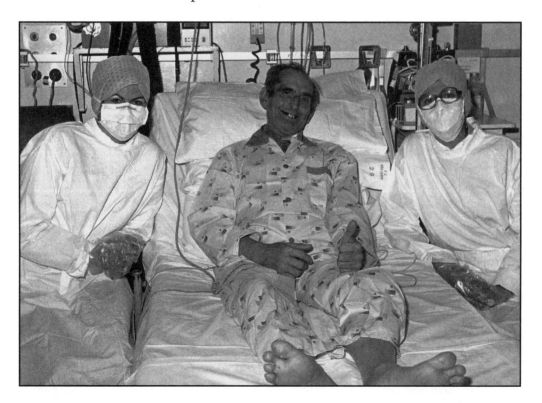

Shumway and his colleagues at Stanford went to work on tackling the problem of rejection. While they did not develop new immunosuppressive medications, they discovered a way of diagnosing early signs of rejection, giving the patient better odds of beating it.

In the early days of transplantation, the risk of infection was so great that elaborate precautions were taken before and after surgery. The patient was kept in an isolated hospital room with an air lock at the entrance. All equipment in the room was carefully cleaned and disinfected, and all attending staff wore caps, masks, overshoes, and sterile gowns. There were constant checks for infection, usually done by swabbing the patient's nose, throat, mouth and other areas and examining the tissue. Any signs of infection were immediately treated with antibiotics. The care was complicated, and the information on infection and rejection not always accurate.

One of Shumway's research assistants, Philip Caves, developed a device called a bioptome, which could obtain a minute portion of the transplanted heart to determine if there were any signs of rejection. The bioptome is a long flexible tube that is inserted into the jugular vein and gently pushed down into the right ventricle of the transplanted heart. Within the bioptome is a small pair of pincers that are able to grab a few tiny pieces of tissue. The tissue is then sent to the lab for analysis. The procedure, known as a biopsy, takes only a few minutes. The patient is not put to sleep but given local anesthesia, which kills pain only in the area being worked upon. Routine biopsies performed with the bioptome can diagnose rejection in its earliest stages, so doctors can adjust the patient's medications to ward off any potential problems. Having first used the bioptome on a patient in 1972, Shumway and his colleagues were pleased with the results. In a medical journal article, they referred to this biopsy method as "rapid and

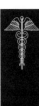

Living Life to Its Fullest

Richard Cope did not exactly fit Norman Shumway's profile for a heart transplant patient; he did not like to follow doctor's orders. But Cope needed and wanted a heart transplant. Forty-five-year-old Cope was a man to go after whatever he wanted, and on October 25, 1970, he became Shumway's twenty-sixth heart transplant patient and a remarkable survivor of the surgery. Three weeks after his operation, he was hiking fifteen miles a day around the hospital. Five weeks after the operation, he went home, where he continued his active lifestyle, playing golf and other sports.

Cope loved being interviewed. As a guest on the *David Frost Show* in 1970, he blurted out the name of the family of his donor heart—Shumway believed keeping the donor family unknown was a way to protect their privacy. In *To Mend the Heart*, Lael Wertenbaker tells the story mostly in Cope's own words. Despite doctors' warnings, Cope traveled whenever and wherever he wanted. "I make sure I have my pills in my hand," he said. Once he even flipped over while riding in a snowmobile. "I thought everyone was going to have a heart attack!" he quipped.

Cope did live through a few episodes of rejection, and the immunosuppressive drugs wreaked havoc on his bones by depleting his body's calcium. He shrank in height from five feet eight inches to five feet five inches and suffered from cracked and broken ribs. Cope recklessly demonstrated that heart transplant survivors can live life to its very fullest. Years after his transplant he said, "I wake up, and it's teeming rain and I hold my face up to it. Hey, what a lousy day? Lousy? Man, if I open my eyes to that day, it's a great day!"

safe, and it is readily accepted as part of the early postoperative routine."[53]

Heart transplant recipient Jim Gleason experienced rejection three months after his operation in 1999. Up until that point he had biweekly biopsies, and no rejection was detected. With each biopsy the dosage of steroids he took was reduced. When his last biopsy showed signs of a problem, his transplant team moved quickly. Within twenty minutes of Gleason's biopsy, a new dosage of steroids—fifty times stronger than his normal daily dosage—was delivered. Gleason was to be on the new dosage for just three days. "I continue to feel great, but then the transplant team always said they would know I was in trouble long before I would ever know of it,"[54] said Gleason. Early detection of rejection by means of myocardial biopsy helps patients avoid serious postoperative complications and maintain normal lives after the transplant.

Heart Transplants No Longer News in the 1970s

While life expectancies for heart transplant recipients gradually increased, media attention for the "medical miracle" procedure faded. By the mid-1970s, heart transplant recipients who survived for a year after their operation had a fifty-fifty chance of surviving another five years; immunosuppressive medication became better understood and better used; myocardial biopsies detected rejection accurately and quickly; and the cost of a heart transplant decreased to only $30,000, about four times the cost for heart valve replacement.

At about this time, heart transplant programs began to standardize techniques, criteria for patients, and donor acceptability. In 1974, Stanford University Medical Center heart transplant patient standards seemed stringent but helped ensure the success of operations. Potential patients should be bedridden or nearly bedridden and given only a six-month prognosis for survival; be under the age of fifty-five; have adequate finances and insurance to cover the cost of pre-transplant evaluation (grant money was available to cover the cost of care at the Stanford hospital); have follow-up medical care available when they returned home; and have a positive attitude with lots of family support. The entire transplant procedure and the risks were discussed with both the patients and their families. Doctors, patients, and patients' families were all better informed to make better decisions throughout the transplant process.

In the first year of heart transplant operations, several surgeons were questioned as to their ethics in finding donors. Even Norman Shumway was investigated by the local district attorney's office about one donor heart. Nothing came of it, but criticism of the

Questions about a Donor's Death

On May 24, 1968, fifty-four-year-old Bruce O. Tucker was brought into the Medical College of Virginia Hospital with a severe head injury. Tucker, an African American factory worker in Richmond, had fallen and hit his head on concrete. After a night at the hospital, doctors determined his situation was hopeless. According to the biography *King of Hearts*, his hospital chart read, "Prognosis for recovery is nil and death imminent." Immediately an effort began to locate Tucker's next of kin. By 2:00 P.M. on May 25, none of Tucker's relatives had been found. Doctors declared him brain-dead and unplugged his respirator. The local medical examiner allowed Richard Lower and his team of transplant surgeons to harvest Tucker's heart and transplant it into forty-eight-year-old Joseph Klett Jr. It was not until after Klett's operation that the hospital medical staff learned that Tucker's brother, William, ran a shoe repair shop just blocks from the medical college.

William Tucker sued the hospital and surgeons for $100,000, claiming white doctors wrongfully took the life of his brother. The Tucker family was represented by L. Douglas Wilder, who later became Virginia's first African American governor. On May 26, 1972, the *Richmond Times Dispatch* reported that Wilder said doctors unplugged Bruce Tucker's respirator not to end his suffering but only because Tucker "was unfortunate enough to come into the hospital at a time when a heart was needed." The defendant's lawyer argued that Tucker was no longer alive even though his heart was beating. The jury sided with Lower, the other doctors, and the hospital, exonerating them.

"Having had an opportunity to discuss the questions in recent months with laymen renewed my faith," that same newspaper reported Lower as saying the next day, after the verdict. "Thoughtful people can come to grips with questions like these and arrive at thoughtful conclusions. . . . This will permit transplantation to continue."

system—or lack of a system—in finding donors was harsh. "It is medically and morally wrong for us as doctors to stand by a dying patient's bedside, hoping he'll get it over with quickly so we can grab his heart,"[55] said Charles Bailey, a pioneer in cardiac surgery.

Denton Cooley countered, saying, "I believe the best way to think of life is that every organ in the body is a servant to the brain. Once the brain is gone the servant is unemployable. Then we must find these organs other employment."[56]

Cooley and those who agreed with him prevailed. In 1974, California passed the Anatomical Gift Act, which permits the removal of a donor heart while it is still beating if there is no evidence of brain function. This made it easier to obtain donor hearts and to transplant them. As Shumway once noted, "No one can transplant a dead heart."[57]

Several positive changes were made in heart transplantation in the 1970s, and by the end of that decade one development ensured even longer survival rates for transplant recipients—a new drug to fight rejection.

Cyclosporine

Rejection is something patients are not even aware of in its early stages. Heart transplant recipient Jim Gleason can only imagine what starts happening in his body during a rejection episode. "Somehow I can picture the red cells saying, 'Hey! That's not our heart—you white cells, go get it! Attack! Protect!' Meanwhile I'm up here looking in telling them all: 'Hey guys, that's a friend keeping us all alive! Make peace, not war!'"[58]

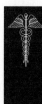

Baby Fae and a Baboon's Heart

On Sunday, October 14, 1984, Baby Fae was born prematurely. A tiny infant with a head full of curly black hair, her underdeveloped heart could not pump enough blood to go around her circulatory system. As a result, her brain, her liver, her kidneys—all her organs—were gradually being starved of oxygen. The situation seemed hopeless.

Then a few days later, Leonard Bailey suggested a way to save Baby Fae. Bailey, a research surgeon at Loma Linda University Medical Center in California, had success transplanting sheep hearts into newborn goats. He had recently been given permission to try his operation on human beings.

Early on the morning of Friday, October 26, 1984, Baby Fae was wheeled into the operating room at Loma Linda where a baboon heart—about the size of a large walnut—was transplanted into her small chest. By 11:35 A.M. the animal's heart began to beat inside the infant. At first it beat too fast, but then it steadied to around 130 beats per minute.

Baby Fae lived for more than two weeks before rejecting the primate's heart. A storm of controversy was played out in the media about the cross-species operation. The debate resulted in the end of animal-to-human transplants for nearly a decade.

Rejection used to be one of the major causes of early death for heart transplant patients. But researchers continued to improve upon the store of antirejection drugs available. One important discovery was cyclosporine, and it had a major impact on the survival rate after all types of organ transplantation. While antirejection drugs are essential for transplant patients' survival, they have serious side effects. They interfere with the immune system's ability to fight off infection, and they can cause bone destruction, weight gain, and damage to arteries. Cyclosporine also kills some immune system cells that fight tumors and reject transplanted organs. However, it does not harm bone marrow cells, which help the body's immune system fight viruses and bacteria that cause infection.

Cyclosporine proved successful in preventing rejection of transplanted pig hearts in laboratory experiments. The British used it for human kidney transplantation in 1978, and it quickly showed a 10 to 20 percent improvement in preventing rejection. It soon became a staple in the fight against heart transplant rejection. Walter Merrill, a heart surgeon at Vanderbilt Medical Center in Nashville, Tennessee, called cyclosporine "a major step forward in reducing the frequency and length of attacks of rejection."[59]

With the development of cyclosporine, cardiac surgeons considered performing more complicated transplant operations.

Heart-Lung Transplants

Experimental heart-lung transplants were performed on dogs as early as 1957 at the University of Mississippi. The dogs lived at most a couple of days. In 1961, researchers at Stanford University did similar experiments with similar results. In 1972, cardiac researcher Aldo Castaneda of Boston had better luck transplanting the hearts and lungs of baboons—many of those lab animals lived as long as six months to a few years. In

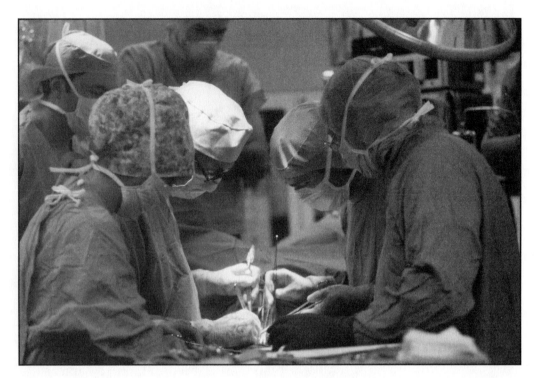

1980, Bruce Reitz at Stanford achieved long-term survival with heart-lung transplants in monkeys.

Human heart-lung transplants were tried by both Cooley and Lillehei in the late 1960s, but their patients survived only a few days. In 1981, Christiaan Barnard tried his hand at the procedure, and his patient survived for twenty-three days.

The first long-term human survivor of a heart-lung transplant had surgery that same year at Stanford. In March 1981, right after the approval of cyclosporine as an immunosuppressive medication in the United States, Bruce Reitz operated on a forty-five-year-old woman with a failing heart caused by high blood pressure in the lungs. The patient, Mary Gohlke, was an advertising executive from Arizona. While the operation was technically successful, recovery was difficult. "My new lungs were working better, but they still hadn't fully expanded. In addition, they still retained some fluid, particularly on the right side,"

Surgeons Bruce Reitz and Norman Shumway attempt a heart-lung transplant on Mary Gohlke, a newspaper executive from Mesa, Arizona.

wrote Gohlke. A drainage tube was inserted into her chest. She said:

> I had been uncomfortable before. Now I couldn't even lie on my right side. My joints, particularly my ankles, swelled from steroids. They were inflamed and it was painful to stand or walk. I didn't mind that part. I didn't feel much like walking anyway. The doctors told us not to worry about the inflammation. It would go away when they were able to reduce the amounts of steroids I was getting.[60]

A serious bout of rejection set in ten days after the transplant. "You see the lungs act like a pump for your kidneys. When your lungs don't work well, neither do your kidneys," said Reitz, Gohlke's surgeon. "In Mary's case, she couldn't breathe well because of the fluid in her lungs, which lowered her kidney function. The lowered kidney function caused more fluid to accumulate in her lungs. It became a vicious cycle until she stopped breathing."[61]

A ventilator tube was inserted in Gohlke's trachea to keep her breathing. When her lungs began to work, so did her kidneys. Her recovery continued without any major problems, and she remained well for several years.

A Viable Alternative

In her book *I'll Take Tomorrow*, Mary Gohlke wrote:

> My life since the transplant operation hasn't been different in some respects from the life of any other person. There are good days and bad ones. There are highs and lows. There are joys and sorrows. Life extracts a certain price. But I can say that I'm truly happy. Although I don't keep up the pace I once did, I have the energy to do many of the things I enjoy: driving, cooking, shopping, entertaining friends, caring for my family. One thing is for certain: if Bruce Reitz came to me and said, 'Mary, something has gone wrong and we're going to have to do another double transplant,' I'd agree to it in a second.[62]

Like countless other transplant survivors, Gohlke believes that trying to hold on to life—even while struggling with problems associated with this operation—is better than letting go.

There are 118 heart transplant programs in the United States, 61 in Europe, and 23 in other parts of the world. According to the Registry of the International Society for Heart Transplantation, 2,450 known heart transplant operations were performed by 1988. Nearly 75 percent of those patients lived at least five years after their surgeries. With the advent of immunosuppressive drugs like cyclosporine, some centers report even better survival statistics.

Improvement in heart transplantation did much to bring it into mainstream medicine. But surgeons now know it is far more than just a simple operation; it is a challenge to monitor and maintain a borrowed heart long after surgery. Aided by myocardial biopsies, the right mix of immunosuppressive medications can be determined for each patient. Those patients in turn must live each day with their new heart by taking care of it, learning how to recognize the signs of trouble, and seeking medical attention immediately. The one element of heart transplantation that cannot be aided and controlled by medical attention is finding a donor. The latest heart transplant research might solve that problem as well.

CHAPTER 5

The Artificial Heart

In the period of euphoria after the first human heart transplant operation, it seemed many people would gladly sign up to donate their organs, including their hearts. In August 1968, when news broke that former president Dwight D. Eisenhower's life was in danger due to serious heart disease, more than twenty people volunteered their own hearts to be transplanted into Eisenhower's failing body. This illustrates that the public in general did not understand the consequences of being a heart donor. In the end it did not matter; neither Eisenhower nor his family even considered heart transplantation as a treatment.

There was no system in place for people to make their hearts available upon their death. For ordinary heart transplant candidates (unlike beloved former presidents), donors were few and far between. During that same period, Houston, Texas, experienced a larger than usual number of accidents and homicides. Still, Denton Cooley could not find many donors.

The situation is much the same today. Even though there is a system in place for both donors and recipients, and people in general are more aware of the importance of organ donation, almost a third of transplant candidates die waiting for a heart to become available.

Unlike other forms of organ transplantation, a life is lost to save another with heart transplantation. Someone has to be declared brain-dead, and often grieving family members must make the difficult decision to authorize the donation. The emotions surrounding such a gift can affect even those who deal with heart transplantation on a regular basis. In his book *Transplant: A Heart Surgeon's Account of the Life and Death Dramas of the New Medicine*, cardiac surgeon and U.S. senator Bill Frist recounts how difficult it was receiving phone calls concerning donors for his wife Karyn. "When I hung up the phone, Karyn was watching me, her big expressive eyes holding a sadness I could never afford to feel. These calls always upset her. I knew she was thinking about the dead man I called a donor, wondering whether he had a wife and children, worrying about how they felt."[63]

Donor hearts always come from patients whose lives cannot be saved—that is the irony and reality of cardiac transplantation. One of the best hopes for solving the shortage of donor hearts has been the development of an artificial heart.

Clash of Texas-Sized Egos

The first surgery implanting an artificial heart into a human being was almost overshadowed by the controversy surrounding it. Medical ethics, medical egos, and research practices were all questioned in the tense atmosphere of a feud between the nation's two most famous cardiac surgeons: Michael DeBakey and Denton Cooley, both of Houston.

Since coming to Texas, DeBakey had reorganized Baylor College of Medicine into a top medical school and research center. In 1968, he became the school's president. It became apparent that DeBakey wanted to top off his achievements by being the first surgeon to develop and implant an artificial heart into a human being.

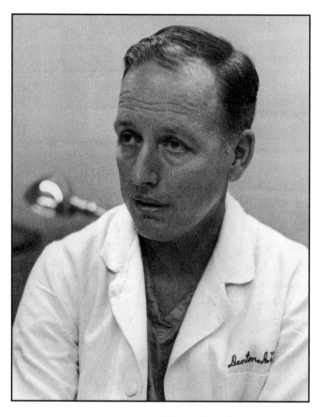

Denton Cooley (pictured) and Michael DeBakey competed for prominence in their field.

Michael DeBakey had become a household name with a reputation no other surgeon could match, with one exception—Denton Cooley. For years the competition for the greatest number of surgeries and the most national attention had put Cooley and DeBakey at odds with one another. To most observers it appeared DeBakey was jealous of Cooley's accomplishments.

In the 1960s, with funding from the National Heart Institute, DeBakey set up a research team to construct an artificial heart. DeBakey had predicted an artificial heart would be ready for implantation in a human by the end of the decade. Later he would up that prediction by another five years. But by September 1968, after five years of building, testing, and starting over again, DeBakey-sponsored researcher Domingo Liotta thought he had made a workable artificial heart.

The trouble was that Liotta could not get DeBakey to okay clinical trials to implant the device in humans. All research, especially that funded by a grant, had to go through official channels before it could be tested. DeBakey had stretched himself so thin with all his obligations that he rarely communicated with the surgeons or researchers he was in charge of. According to one Houston doctor,

> Every time Domingo finally got through to Mike to urge that more attention be paid to the artificial heart, he would be told to get back down to the laboratory and continue his work. Mike keeps his eye on people and

their work in his own way. But there were weeks, sometimes months, when Liotta couldn't get through to Mike
at all. He began to feel DeBakey was simply not interested in the artificial heart.[64]

Liotta became frustrated. In December 1968, he met
with Houston's other famous surgeon, Denton
Cooley, to talk over his dilemma. Cooley sympa-
thized with Liotta and offered him an alternative. On
April 4, 1969, Denton Cooley, with Domingo Liotta
assisting him, became the first surgeon to implant an
artificial heart into a human being. The mechanism
was attached just like a donor heart in heart transplantation and connected by two polyethylene tubes
to a control console about the size of a large filing cabinet. The patient was forty-seven-year-old Haskell
Karp, a printing estimator from Illinois. Karp was
restricted to lying in bed or sitting in a chair to remain
connected to the large console.

*Haskell Karp lies on
his bed after receiving
a totally mechanical
heart on April 4, 1969.*

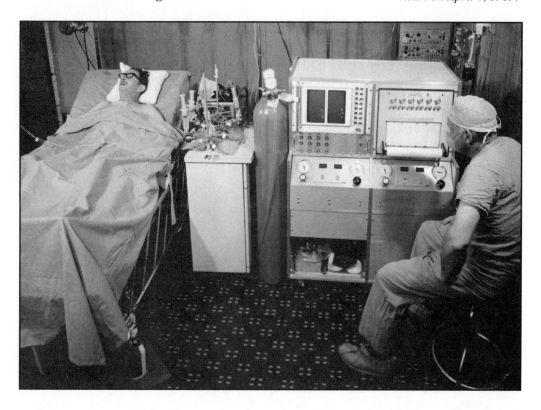

The morning of April 5, 1969, Cooley announced his latest feat to the world. While making an appeal for a donor heart, Cooley explained the surgery was a stopgap measure to keep Haskell alive long enough to receive a heart transplant. Karp survived for sixty-three days with the artificial heart before having it replaced with a donor heart from a forty-year-old woman. Less than twenty-four hours after his heart transplant, Karp died.

DeBakey did not learn about the first artificial heart implantation until he was questioned at a meeting of the National Heart Institute a day after the operation. Embarrassed about not being informed and angry about having the limelight stolen from him, DeBakey went on the defensive, charging Cooley with unethical behavior: "Application of an unproved device . . . into a human being for primary experimentation before its safety and effectiveness had been proved scientifically in animal experiments is a breach of scientific ethics."[65]

The National Heart Institute launched an investigation into the incident. The first thing DeBakey noticed was that the device Cooley implanted into Karp looked very much like the one Liotta had been working on for him. Liotta said it was different. Cooley maintained that Liotta began working on the implanted mechanism in his free time on nights and weekends. Cooley had given Liotta $20,000 to come up with a separate device from DeBakey's.

Cooley was also asked why he did not keep DeBakey informed of his work with Liotta. Cooley replied, "Having met with nothing but negative replies to anything of this nature, and being determined to develop this device, we did not make a formal report." In further defense of himself, Cooley told reporters: "I have done more heart surgery than anyone else in the world. Based on this experience, I believe I am qualified to judge what is right and proper for my patients. The permission I receive to do

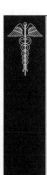

Widow Has a Change of Heart

The press coverage surrounding Denton Cooley's historic surgery on Haskell Karp affected everyone involved. Shirley Karp began questioning her decision, her husband's decisions, and Denton Cooley's motivations shortly after her husband's death. She wondered whether or not Cooley's operation on her husband was a good idea. As time went on, she became well aware of all the criticism leveled against Cooley for the surgery.

Shirley Karp called Cooley and asked if the artificial heart had been properly tested and if Cooley had stolen it as the newspapers had reported. Cooley tried to assure her he had done everything possible to save her husband's life and that her husband had wanted the operation. But Cooley's words did not appease her.

In April 1971, Shirley Karp brought a $4.5 million malpractice suit against Denton Cooley and Domingo Liotta. Although she had signed a release for her husband's surgery and afterward publicly praised Cooley, she claimed in her suit that she did not understand what she was signing. In Minetree's biography of Cooley, she is quoted as saying that her husband was "the unfortunate victim of human experimentation." She further claimed that neither she nor her husband knew that the artificial heart had never been used in a human being. Fortunately for Cooley, her malpractice suit was dismissed in July 1972.

what I do, I receive from my patients. It is not received from a government agency or from one of my seniors."[66]

Cooley took all the official blame for the incident, but his surgical practice and reputation survived intact. The interest in the artificial heart died by 1970 along with the interest in heart transplantation. As cardiologist Jim Nora put it: "It ended with a whimper, not a bang."[67] But it would be revived later.

Early Artificial Heart Research

The idea of an artificial heart for human beings has been around even longer than the idea of heart transplantation. The development of medical devices like the pacemaker, artificial heart valves, the heart-lung machine, and pump oxygenators all preceded and influenced different versions of the artificial heart.

In 1937, Russian Vladimir Demikhov designed an artificial heart approximately the size of a normal heart. The device had two pumps side by side filled with saline solution. Demikhov implanted the mechanism into three dogs that year and five more in 1938. One dog survived as long as five and a half hours. Demikhov did not think his device could maintain the life of a human being, but he did think it could maintain the organs of a dead donor before a transplantation operation.

At Japan's Tokyo University School of Medicine, two artificial hearts were developed by a research team led by Yukihiko Atsumi. In 1958, their hydraulically driven plastic heart maintained a dog's heartbeat for up to six hours. Two years later a roller pump

The Pioneering Aviator and the Pioneering Surgeon

Charles Lindbergh was perhaps the most famous man of his time. Lindbergh made the first solo nonstop flight across the Atlantic Ocean in 1927. A shy man who never sought the media attention he received, Lindbergh was often inspired by the people closest to him. He grew very concerned about his sister-in-law, who suffered from rheumatic heart disease. Doctors did not offer her any hope. Lindbergh wondered whether surgery could help her. He began thinking about developing some kind of mechanical pump that could take over for her heart while surgeons operated.

After meeting Lindbergh in New York, heart researcher Alexis Carrell became interested in the aviator's design for what was thought of at the time as an "artificial heart." Carrell created a device using Lindbergh's ideas.

Although it was never used to help Lindbergh's sister-in-law, Carrell successfully used it to preserve hearts, spleens, kidneys, and pancreases for experimental surgery. The mechanism is credited with laying the groundwork for the development of heart-lung machines and the artificial heart.

Charles Lindbergh experimented with designs for an artificial heart pump.

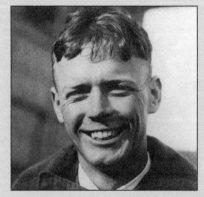

powered by a miniature motor supported an animal for thirteen hours. The Japanese machines had problems with blood clots causing blockage in the arteries. They tried lining the pump with silicone rubber and managed to keep a dog alive for twenty-seven hours. Still, most of their lab animals died from blocked arteries.

In the United States, Willem Kolff, who had designed an artificial kidney, also worked on an artificial heart. In 1959, working with Japanese engineers Tetsuzo Akutsu and Yukihiko Nose, his team implanted a pendulum type of artificial heart into a dog. One side of the pump filled up as the other side emptied. The dog's blood pressure remained normal for five hours as the ventricles of this pump emptied alternately. By 1965, they designed a one-piece, four-chamber heart and implanted it into a calf, which lived for thirty-one hours. After heart transplantation became a reality, Kolff concentrated on developing short-term support for patients awaiting donor organs.

Partial Artificial Hearts

Not all implantable devices replace hearts; some only assist them. A left ventricle assist device (LVAD) is a partial artificial heart that boosts the left ventricle's pumping action. In 1963, Stanley Crawford, a member of DeBakey's surgical team, implanted an LVAD into a forty-two-year-old, brain-damaged man who was also facing severe heart failure. The mechanism was developed by a group of researchers DeBakey assembled that included Domingo Liotta. The LVAD was attached to the left side of the patient's heart and hooked up to a large external console. It kept the man's heart beating normally for four days until he was declared brain-dead.

While DeBakey worked on perfecting the LVAD, Dwight Harken in Boston explored another concept. Harken designed a pump to improve the blood flow through the body. Harken's pump moved blood from the aorta during the heart's contractions and pumped it back into circulation when the heart relaxed. As a result, more blood flowed when the heart relaxed.

Harken's pump was an external device in which the exchange of blood took place through a tube inserted into the aorta. In 1966, DeBakey used Harken's machine on a sixty-five-year-old coal miner with rheumatic mitral stenosis to wean him from cardiopulmonary bypass after heart surgery. The pump sat next to the patient's bedside and maintained the patient's blood flow for several days, but unfortunately it was not enough to save his life.

Later that year DeBakey succesfully used the LVAD on a thirty-seven-year-old woman suffering from heart failure. It supported the patient's heart for ten days until the heart could sustain itself. Then the LVAD was removed. Eighteen days later the woman went home from the hospital healthy.

By the 1970s, interest in the total artificial heart began to grow again. Artificial heart programs popped up in a dozen laboratories worldwide in countries like Argentina, Austria, China, Czechoslovakia, France, Germany, Italy, Japan, Russia, and the United States. But a mechanical heart developed in Utah captured the world's attention.

The Jarvik Heart

The son of a physician, Robert Jarvik grew up with a talent

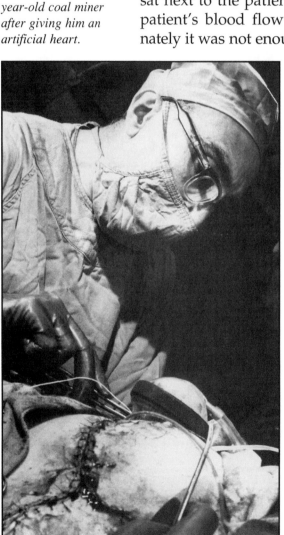

Michael DeBakey finishes closing the chest of a sixty-five-year-old coal miner after giving him an artificial heart.

for design and engineering. As a teenager he devised improvements to his father's surgical equipment. He began studying architecture in college, later switching to medicine. In 1970, Jarvik joined the University of Utah's Institute for Biomedical Engineering, where a program to design an artificial heart was being conducted.

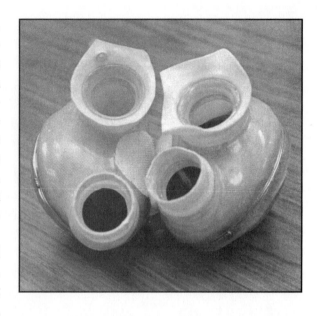

Jarvik developed several artificial heart prototypes, always improving on his last model. Finally, the Jarvik 7, made to conform to the human body, sustained the life of a calf it was implanted in for 221 days. The young animal grew in size beyond the capacity for which the device was constructed.

The Jarvik 7 artificial heart was used to keep patient Barney Clark alive for 112 days.

The Jarvik 7 consisted of two ventricles made of polyurethane on an alumimum base that was implanted in the laboratory animal. The device was air-driven and required a dishwasher-sized pump to make it work.

In January 1981, Jarvik made some predictions about the artificial heart. "How long will it be before total artificial hearts are routinely implanted in human beings? Probably at least a decade although clinical trials on a small scale may begin sooner." Jarvik believed in the possibility of the artificial heart, but he was not naive. Though his latest version was an improvement over earlier models, Jarvik understood its limitations:

> Why then will it be so long before artificial hearts are routinely implanted? The answer is to be found mainly in ethical considerations and in the allocation of the limited money available for research on the artificial heart.

The pneumatically powered hearts that have proved successful in animals are not portable. The animal is confined to a cage, tethered to a large drive system and exercised only on a treadmill. Such conditions would be unacceptable for human beings.[68]

The Jarvik 7 could not be viewed as a permanent, life-saving device, but it was about to be used in just that fashion.

Barney Clark's Last Days

Barney Clark was a sixty-two-year-old retired dentist from Seattle. He had smoked cigarettes most of his life, developing several serious conditions that damaged his heart and lungs. Because of his medical history, Clark was not a candidate for conventional heart transplantation. While in the hospital, Clark told his nurses why he gave up fishing: "I cannot stand seeing the fish gasping for breath on the dock, like I do." When shown the calves implanted with Jarvik 7s, he commented, "These calves cannot speak, but I believe they feel a lot better than I do."[69]

In December 1982, surgeon William De Vries implanted the Jarvik 7 into Barney Clark. The more than seven-hour operation was difficult. The size of the Jarvik 7 and the series of tubes and lines running from the patient to the controller unit made it impossible to close Clark's chest. When the pump was started, there

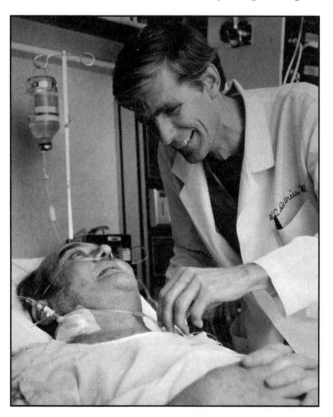

Artificial heart recipient Barney Clark smiles up at Dr. William De Vries the day after his history-making operation.

was a problem with one of the valves. It was quickly replaced. Despite the difficulties, the mechanical heart began working for Clark and kept him alive for 112 days. But life with the Jarvik 7 was anything but comfortable. The number of tubes connecting it to the 350-pound controller kept Clark in bed and his body more susceptible to infection. Clark drifted in and out of consciousness, suffering from a series of complications including epileptic convulsions, lung problems, kidney failure, and pneumonia. Throughout the ordeal Clark maintained a sense of humor.

The public was fascinated by Clark's surgery, and to satisfy that fascination the media would do just about anything to get the story. One reporter even sneaked inside the hospital in a laundry cart. Enthusiasm for the artificial heart waned as more reports of Clark's condition surfaced along with the cost of the experiment. More than $160 million had been invested in the Jarvik 7 clinical trials, most of it from the federal government, which spearheaded the development of the artificial heart.

William Schroeder survived the longest with an implanted Jarvik 7—620 days—but like Clark he was ill and uncomfortable. He suffered several strokes and infections.

In the 1980s, public expectations for the artificial heart were high. The cost, as well as the suffering the Jarvik 7 recipients endured, lowered those expectations. Both the public and the media questioned the need for such a device. It was as if researchers and surgeons did not heed Robert Jarvik's warning about the limited technology, high expectations, and quality-of-life issues associated with the artificial heart. For the next decade most mechanical cardiac-assist efforts concentrated on developing and refining "bridges to transplantation" like the LVAD. In September 1985, the Jarvik 7 was used as a successful bridge to transplantation for twenty-five-year-old Michael Drummond. A viral disease had attacked Drummond's heart, and nine days after the implantation of the Jarvik 7 a donor heart became available. It was successfully transplanted into Drummond.

According to David Lederman, developer of the latest mechanical heart, the portable AbioCor, the clinical trials of the Jarvik 7 "set this field back at least 10 or 15 years." Lederman and his company, Abiomed, learned from the Jarvik 7 experience. "It was a public relations disaster, but it was a very important first step," said Lederman. "We knew in 1982 that the expectations of the public at large were of a technology that was impossible to meet."[70] Lederman invested two decades of work into the development of a better artificial heart—one a recipient can truly live with.

The AbioCor at the Dawn of the New Century

"Every step we did was really a new adventure for us,"[71] said Lamon Gray Jr. of the historic surgery that took place on July 2, 2001, at Jewish Hospital in Louisville, Kentucky.

"The operation was very difficult, it was long but it was also kind of a thing of beauty,"[72] said Rob D. Dowling.

Both Gray and Dowling were part of a team of fourteen surgeons, nurses, anesthesiologists, and other support staff that implanted the AbioCor artificial heart into fifty-nine-year-old Robert Tools of Franklin, Kentucky. Before the operation, Tools was diagnosed with severe end-stage heart failure. In 1992, he suffered two heart attacks and had quadruple bypass surgery. In 1995, he developed congestive heart failure and diabetes. He was evaluated for heart transplantation late in 1998 at St. Thomas Hospital in Nashville, Tennessee, where he was determined to be unsuitable for the operation due to his other health problems. By the summer of 2001, doctors expected Tools to live no more than thirty days. If all went well, the device would not only extend Tools's survival but improve his quality of life.

Unlike the artificial hearts of the past, the AbioCor was designed to fit inside the body without any tubes or wires connecting it to an external pump or power source. Patients do not have to remain in bed; they can resume a relatively normal lifestyle. Internal batteries can operate the heart for one-half hour—for taking a shower, for example. An external battery pack that provides long-term power, depending on the number

His Life a Milestone in Medical History

When Robert Tools came to after having an artificial heart implanted inside him, he announced to the world that he was happy to be awake, seeing people around him and knowing that he was alive. Those watching the development of the latest artificial heart could not have agreed with Tools more.

Born in Mobile, Alabama, Tools worked most of his life for the telephone company in the South and the Midwest. When he was diagnosed with severe end-stage heart failure in 2001, he became interested in the AbioCor study. He proved to be a great candidate for clinical trials.

David Lederman, Abiomed's chief executive officer, reflected upon his relationship with Tools, in a November 2001 Jewish Hospital press release. "Bob Tools was an extraordinarily courageous man," Lederman was quoted as saying, "Everyone who came in contact with him was impressed by his strength of spirit, his wit and intelligence and by the resolve with which he fought to survive." Lederman remembered after the operation asking Tools if he could feel his heart beating.

Tools said no. Later when a reporter asked Tools if the AbioCor made any noise, Tools replied that it whirs. Concerned, Lederman wanted to know why Tools never told him of the sound. "You didn't ask me if I hear a sound," said Tools, and besides, Tools added, he liked the noise because it told him his heart was working.

Robert Tools grasps a model of the AbioCor replacement heart at Jewish Hospital in Louisville, Kentucky.

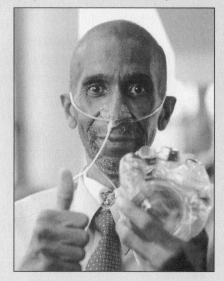

of batteries carried, can be worn next to the body. An energy transfer device enables the batteries to power the pump without being directly connected to it.

Tools's operation continued for more than seven hours. The surgical team remained cautious with each individual procedure. "This was really the first time we ever implanted it into a human and we weren't sure it was going to fit," said Gray. It did fit, and the excitement level in the operating room was high. "The room was just full of energy. I can remember thinking 'Boy this is really cool! This is really neat that everyone just pulled together!'" said Dowling. "I would think of something I needed and Bam it would be in my hand."[73]

The time came to switch on the artificial heart. There was no turning back. "We disconnected all the external power and now we had Mr. Tools pumping with his artificial heart on his internal battery that had absolutely no connection to the outside world," said Gray. "I mean this is the first time this has happened and it sends shivers up your spine. It was truly a thrilling moment."[74]

Tools's new man-made heart kept beating and kept Robert Tools alive for nearly five months. His death was unrelated to the implantation of the artificial heart or to a stroke he suffered after the July 2 operation but to abdominal bleeding brought on by his preexisting medical conditions. "These patients are the sickest of the sick," said Gray of those involved in the AbioCor clinical trials. "They will die in a very short time without some kind of intervention and their families understand the risks of the surgery, and the risks of no further intervention. It takes a great deal of courage to agree to take a step that no one else has taken."[75] To Gray and the staff at Jewish Hospital, the clinical trial patients are heroes.

Abiomed is only one of several companies developing artificial hearts. The current artificial heart clinical trials are being carefully observed by heart doctors and researchers around the world. The implanted AbioCors were expected to extend clinical trial participants' lives by only thirty to sixty days. As of May 2002, those expectations have been exceeded by most of the artificial heart recipients in the six medical centers involved. The second artificial heart recipient, Tom Christerson, even returned home and is living a relatively normal, healthy life. The trial results look encouraging for the future of the artificial heart and for those seeking an alternative to heart transplantation in the battle against the nation's number one killer, heart disease.

Tools's wife, Carol, said in the same report that her husband was glad to participate in the clinical trials. "He has been able to make a difference for mankind, enjoy some of his favorite things in life, and experience a bit of notoriety—and for Bob, nothing could have been better."

CHAPTER 6

Now and the Future

A life can change in an instant. Gordon Milby is proof of that. As a high school principal and former coach, Milby always took good care of himself; he ate right and exercised regularly. In 1995, most people would have described Milby at age forty-nine as the picture of health. But unknown to Milby, something was seriously wrong with his heart. "I became very sick in July 1995, while on a trip to Florida," explained Milby. "When I returned to Kentucky I checked with my doctor and at that time he put me on medication and tried to help my failing heart. The diagnosis was cardiomyopathy. I was told that someday I would need a heart transplant."[76] For a while medication worked for Milby. Then, on the evening after his first day of school, he became ill. His wife found him on the floor turning blue. He was rushed to the local hospital and then transferred to Jewish Hospital in Louisville.

While heart transplantation is no longer experimental, it is still the treatment of last resort—a treatment used when all else has failed. In 1995, Milby was at that point. "I was reevaluating my whole life," he said. "It really makes you stop and notice the important things like your family and the quality of your life together." Most of all Milby thought about his oldest grandson, who has cerebral palsy. "I knew I had to fight to be here with him,"[77] he said. So Milby came home to Louisville, Kentucky, and began his fight for life by waiting for a donor.

Bridges to Transplantation

On November 17, 1995, Gordon Milby was told he had less than twenty-four hours to live. His doctors at Jewish Hospital asked if he would like to join an experimental program and be a patient in clinical trials for a left ventricle assist device (LVAD) developed by the Baxter Company in California. Doctors hoped the device could keep Milby alive until a donor heart became available. "There was not much of a choice to be made! My family and I made the decision to have the device implanted in me to help me survive until I could receive a heart transplant,"[78] said Milby. The pump was surgically implanted in Milby that same day, his oldest grandson's birthday.

Left ventricle assist devices such as this one have been used to sustain countless lives.

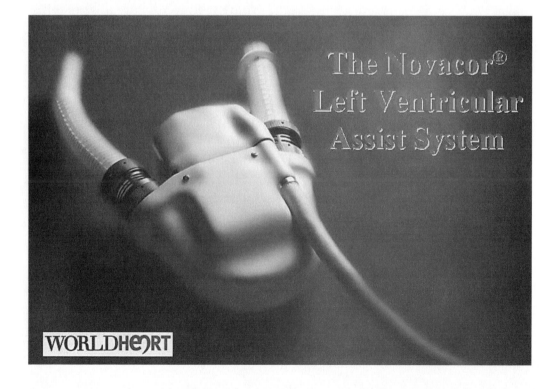

The Novacor® Left Ventricular Assist System

WORLDHEART

LVADs and similar mechanical pumps are sometimes incorrectly called artificial hearts. They do not take the place of a diseased or damaged heart; they only assist the heart, boosting the left ventricle's pumping action. LVADs and ventricle assist devices (VADs) are surgically implanted around the ventricles, "piggybacking" the heart. "There are between three and four thousand heart transplants done in the world every year total. The number has not increased in the last ten years and probably won't unless some other source of donor organs arises," said Stanford cardiologist Randall Vagelos regarding the need for these devices. "Considering that there are 400,000 new cases of heart failure in our country alone annually, it is clear that the current options for treatment of end-stage heart failure are insufficient."[79]

LVADs and VADs can help without seriously changing a heart patient's lifestyle, but some adjustments have to be made. "Any signs of redness, I had to call my doctors," said Milby about the area where his LVAD connected to its external batteries. "I had to constantly keep it clean." The external batteries of Milby's LVAD lasted three hours, with a forty-five-minute spare battery. The closest Milby ever came to running his batteries too low was when he attended a wedding. When he came home, he had only ten to fifteen minutes left on the spare battery. "That was cutting it close; too close really," said Milby. At first the noise the LVAD made irritated Milby, but he got used to it. "In fact, I kind of missed it after my transplant,"[80] he said.

The mechanical pump cannot completely solve a diseased heart's problems. Milby's heart needed some additional help. For a short period of time a defibrillator was implanted into Milby's chest because even with the LVAD his heart had a tendency to skip a beat. "It was almost like a short in a car," said Milby. "It just shocked my heart back into rhythm when I needed it."[81]

More research and development is being done on a variety of temporary mechanical heart pumps. For example, some smaller VADs in development can provide continuous blood flow without the pulsing action of the natural heart. But the heart's pulsing action keeps blood cells from building up in diseased and narrowed arteries—the accumulation of blood cells can cause clots that can lead to strokes. This drawback to the nonpulsative VADs will have to be overcome by researchers.

LVADs cannot be used on hearts that have both the left and right ventricles damaged. In chronic heart failure, eventually both ventricles stop functioning. However, biventricular assist devices are available for heart patients. For instance, the BVS 2000 is a biventricular support system and "bridge" device that assumes the heart's pumping action for both the left and right ventricles, allowing the heart to rest and heal itself. The BVS is used to help patients recover from open-heart surgery, maintain a working heart

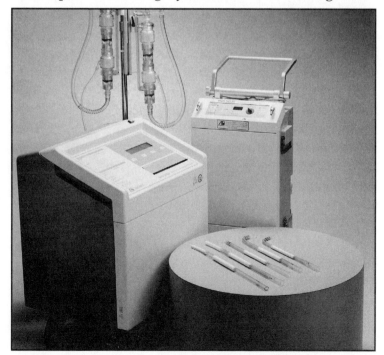

The BVS 2000 provides short-term support for failing but recoverable hearts.

until transplantation, and assist newly transplanted hearts. Vagelos believes these temporary pumps could be beneficial for more patients in the future.

Research to develop new and better ventricle assist devices seems a logical next step in combating heart failure. Currently, LVADs and VADs are very expensive. Vagelos says if the cost and the risk or complications of these devices come down, more of them will be used:

> Whether these devices will become safe enough, and then whether our society is interested in investing in these devices, are huge economic and social issues. You might say that since a good percentage of all the people who die in this country die from heart disease, everyone should be entitled to the possible life-extending attributes of mechanical cardiac support. On the other hand, I'm not sure that anyone is interested in really thinking that globally in terms of expanding our life span.[82]

Gordon Milby avoided the cost of the implantation of his LVAD because he was part of an experimental study. Milby's LVAD managed to keep him alive for 217 days until a donor heart was found, but not without complications. Besides having a defibrillator implanted, Milby had two lung surgeries. "I thought I was going to lose a lung but I didn't,"[83] said Milby. He remained in intensive care for a month. Then he was moved to a transitional unit where he began physical therapy (in his case, exercising and bicycling) on a regular basis. Milby had lost a lot of weight and had to build himself up while waiting for a heart.

The Need for Family Support

On June 21, 1996, Gordon Milby received a fifteen-year-old heart. He spent only five days in the hospital recovering from his transplant surgery. Eight days after the operation, he was back to work as principal of Doss High School in Louisville, Kentucky.

Milby said in an interview that he had been glad the long wait was finally over: "Two hundred seventeen days! Now I have a better idea of what women go through having babies," said Milby. "This was my baby! The excitement and joy of that phone call [saying he had a donor heart] can never be explained and can never be replaced." It was not long before Milby's joy was increased by the reality of being a heart transplant recipient. "I knew I could never look back."[84]

While Milby does not recall any long-term depression after his operation, he did feel sad about the donor. "It depressed me that someone else had to die for me to live—I felt the pain they were feeling," said Milby. "What made it easier for me was that I found out the

First Family-Shared Heart

Parents give their children life, and children generally outlive their parents. That is the rule for most families. A dramatic exception to this rule occurred in late August 1994.

Chester Szuber, a retired Michigan Christmas-tree-farm owner, had been on a waiting list for a donor heart for four years when news came that one was finally available. The donor heart belonged to a twenty-two-year-old nursing student named Patti who was declared brain-dead after an automobile accident in the Great Smoky Mountains National Park. She had taken a vacation there before the college semester began. Patti carried a donor card; she had informed her family about her decision and even had a bumper sticker on her car promoting organ donation. As it happened, Patti was Chester Szuber's youngest child.

While the idea of transplanting her daughter's heart into her dying husband was difficult for Jeanne Szuber, Chester insisted. In a September 5, 1994, article in *Time*, he said, "It would be a joy to have Patti's heart." The rest of the Szuber family agreed, and within six hours Patti's heart was flown back to Michigan and transplanted into her father. Released two weeks later from William Beaumont Hospital, in Royal Oaks, Michigan, Chester Szuber was proud to have his daughter's heart beating inside him.

According to Joel Newman, spokesman for the United Network for Organ Sharing, this was the first time a heart was transplanted from one family member to another, clearly illustrating the need for more organ donations. "While the odds of this occurring are extremely slim, this puts a human face on a real problem for thousands of people awaiting organs," Newman was quoted as saying in that same *Time* article. "You can save lives by donating."

donor's family was glad their son's heart went to a high school principal—someone who helps others."[85]

A transplant patient's attitude is critically important. "It is hard to be a transplant recipient, as it is difficult for anyone with a chronic illness," said Dr. Darla Granger, a transplant rejection specialist at Jewish Hospital in Louisville, Kentucky. "Sometimes being 'well' is even more difficult—you have to remember to keep taking your medicines on a regularly scheduled basis even when you don't feel 'sick' because otherwise you will reject your organ."[86]

Milby was lucky to have a good attitude and a strong support system of family and friends: "I don't know what I would have done without my wife, my two daughters and two sons in law, my golfing buddies and my two doctors,"[87] he said.

"We insist that potential recipients have a support person because there will be days you want to give up and it is important to have someone around who will remind you why you want to live," said Granger. "People who do not want to live will die. Transplant psychiatrists are an integral part of the transplant team."[88]

Before the transplant, Milby says there were good days and bad ones. "I knew I had to fight to survive." Sometimes the wait was even more difficult for his wife. "We just tried to take it a day at a time," said Milby. "On those bad days, I'd just hold my wife and let her cry until she felt better—we just made the best of it, that's all we could do." That perseverance helped Milby since his transplant as well. Three years after the operation, Milby's wife suffered a brain aneurysm and died suddenly. "It was a shock because she was in much better shape and our focus had been on getting and keeping me well."[89]

Anxiety about every setback after a transplant is common. Change is hard on everyone, and the changes transplant recipients go through affect not only them but everyone around them. Understanding the risks and the changes transplantation brings to a recipient's life often makes it easier to deal with. "Life has to go on," said Milby. "I have been blessed with four more grandchildren since my transplant." Milby has also remarried and retired. One of the things he enjoys most about his life now is volunteering at Jewish Hospital. "I now help other people going through transplants understand what will happen to them and how they can cope,"[90] said Milby. For Milby, helping others makes a positive difference for them and him.

Coping with Rejection Today

An organ transplant is much more than an operation. Surgeons are only part of the team of medical professionals guiding the patient through the transplant ordeal. "We've gotten much better at treating patients for the long term, after an organ transplant," said Walter Merrill, a heart surgeon at Vanderbilt University. "And it is in that aftercare—especially treating rejection—where most of the work really is."[91] Patients cannot benefit from surgery without skillful care and monitoring after an organ transplant.

According to Granger, rejection is both more common and more serious in heart transplants than with some other organs. For example, kidney recipients can go on dialysis if their transplanted organ fails. "It clearly is more serious because like liver-transplant recipients, they must keep their organ to survive," said Granger of heart recipients. "Livers can regenerate, unlike hearts, so even in liver transplant recipients rejection is less dangerous than in heart recipients."[92]

"I will live with the possibility of having a rejection episode for the rest of my life," says Gordon Milby.[93] While the risk of rejection decreases with time, it is always an issue. As long as he lives, Milby will take antirejection medication and be checked regularly for early signs of rejection. When blood tests indicate rejection, biopsies are usually done to confirm the

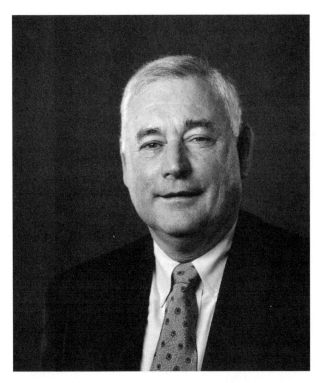

Gordon Milby is one long-term survivor of heart transplant surgery.

result. Milby has been very lucky; as recently as May 2002, he has had only one questionable blood sample that needed to be checked further. His doctors made a slight change in his medication, and he was fine again.

In the past two decades, several new drugs have been developed that help doctors better treat transplant patients for rejection. Unfortunately, most of these immunosuppressives still produce serious side effects. Some impair kidney function, some increase cholesterol levels, and some are hard on bones, making them soft, weak, and prone to fractures. Many heart transplant recipients, including Gordon Milby, have to have their bones scanned a few times a year to check for any weakness.

Some medications can change patients' moods, creating either irritability or euphoria. Occasionally, the psychological effects of the antirejection drug are severe enough for doctors to recommend medication to counteract its side effects. New drugs and treatments are constantly being evaluated.

A new kind of light therapy has been successful in reducing the risk of transplant rejection. Called photophoresis, the technique uses light to destroy blood cells that cause organ rejection. In this process, blood is pumped from the patient's body and then white blood cells in that blood are treated with ultraviolet light and a chemical that makes the cells very sensitive to the light. Finally, the blood is returned to the patient's body. This method has not been proven to increase a transplant patient's lifespan, but it has helped limit the amount of antirejection drugs recipients need.

Because antirejection drugs weaken the immune system, it is very difficult to deal with infection and rejection at the same time. Perhaps the best treatment for rejection is a combination of medication, education, and communication. All doctors and dentists who treat transplant recipients must be informed of the medications they are taking. "To be successful as a transplant recipient, knowledge is an important thing. I always tell recipients that I went into transplant surgery to work with them to get better—it truly is a partnership," said Granger. "The medication affects each person differently; it is important for the recipient to understand what their medications are doing both to them and for them. It is important for the recipient to know their history and how they responded to [drugs] . . . in the past."[94]

Expanding Eligibility

Heart surgeon Walter Merrill believes the growth in the number of transplant survivors is in part a result of how donors and recipients are being chosen. "We do a much better job of finding appropriate donors and picking out likely recipients than we ever did in the past,"[95] said Merrill. Improvements in rejection therapy, preserving donor organs, and patient support have contributed to an expansion of eligibility for heart transplantaton.

There are more than one hundred different places in the United States where patients can receive heart transplants. Each has its own criteria, but generally patients who are currently smoking cigarettes or abusing drugs or alcohol are not thought of as good transplant candidates. A former smoker or recovering addict or alcoholic could be considered. A candidate cannot have active cancer or any serious active infections. An obese person might be put on a transplant

list, but because that person would need a much larger size heart, the chances of getting a donor are remote.
But perhaps the most important quality a transplant
candidate needs is motivation to get well—those who
will take the necessary medications, persevere during
setbacks, and maintain a positive attitude about the
procedure. Some candidates find their motivation by
being part of a transplant support group.

Potential candidates undergo a series of physical
and psychological tests to see if a heart transplant is
the right treatment for them. Once they are recom-
mended for the procedure, they are put on an organ
donor waiting list. They should be within two to
three hours of the hospital, although some institu-
tions will transport patients by air ambulance.
Sometimes this means a patient has to relocate during
the waiting period. The hospital typically gives the
candidate a beeper so they can be reached anytime to
let them know a donor heart has become available.
By law, heart transplants are done on a first come,
first served basis, with the possible exception of those
that become so ill they must be hospitalized in intensive care. The recipient and donor's blood types must
also match.

Despite the restrictions for candidates, more and
more people are now eligible for cardiac transplantation. "The rule used to be, recipients have to be under 60
years of age," said Merrill. "Now it is not unusual for
patients well into their 60s to have a heart transplant."[96]

The Future of the Artificial Heart

David Lederman believes that his company's artificial heart will be available to American surgeons on a
regular basis sometime in 2004. Seven patients had
the AbioCor implanted in them during the first year
of clinical trials. All of those patients were expected to
survive less than thirty days at the time of their
experimental surgeries. Only two of those recipients
are alive. Three died of strokes possibly resulting

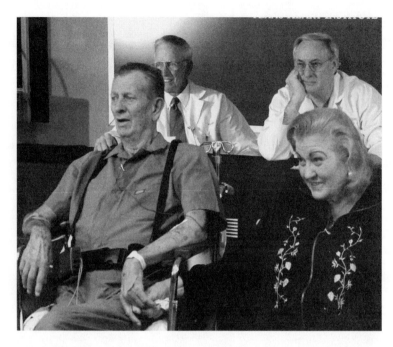

*AbioCor recipient
Bobby Harrison
gathers with his family
to answer questions at
a press conference.*

from blood clots developed in and around the AbioCor. Retired firefighter Bobby Harrison was one of those recipients. "It was a bitter pill for us," said Texas Heart Institute transplant surgeon O. H. Frazier about Harrison's death. "But he was unable to tolerate a full dose of anticoagulant drugs. If he could have, I'm sure he would be alive today."[97]

AbioCor clinical trials were suspended for a short period while the artificial heart design was adjusted to lessen the clotting problem; then the trials started again. It is estimated the implanted AbioCors have beat 1.5 billion times in the trial recipients without one mechanical malfunction. "When the software geniuses at Microsoft design a new program, they can't claim that kind of reliability," said Rob Dowling of the early success of the AbioCor.

Abiomed is working on developing a smaller version of the mechanical heart. "We are also investing significantly in the so-called Penn State heart, a smaller replacement device that is based on a technology developed at Pennsylvania State University,"[99] said Lederman.

Inspiration Taken to Heart

David Lederman grew up in Colombia, South America. The first time he came to the United States was to study aerospace engineering at Cornell University in Ithaca, New York. In 1968, however, a speaker at Cornell changed Lederman's life and career.

Arthur Kantrowitz, a renowned physicist whose work ranged from outside the earth's atmosphere to inside the body, proved that reentry from outer space was possible and invented the first successful heart-assist device. Kantrowitz had taught engineering at Cornell and in 1968 was working on building an artificial heart for Avco Corporation. In 2002, Kenneth Aaron interviewed both Lederman and Kantrowitz for *Cornell Engineering Magazine*. In the interview Lederman recalled his first encounter with Kantrowitz. "He gave a talk on what people who have studied fluid mechanics could do to advance the development of devices and technologies that help the failing heart and replace the failing heart," said Lederman, who was so moved by Kantrowitz's speech that he took the physicist to dinner and then asked him for a job.

"I asked him if he was interested in more than a job—asked him if he was interested in a lifelong career," Kantrowitz, now a professor emeritus at Dartmouth College, said in the interview. Lederman wanted that lifelong career. When he finished his doctorate in 1973, he went to work for Avco. Later Lederman founded Abiomed Inc. in Danvers, Massachusetts, the company that made the first portable, totally implantable artificial heart.

"He was the best chance, by far," said Kantrowitz. "You could see that he had a lot of drive and you could see that he was a very intelligent person."

Under Lederman's leadership, Abiomed has found an important niche in the competitive medical research marketplace. In 2001, the company's artificial heart, the AbioCor, was named technology of the year by *Industry Week* and invention of the year by *Time* magazine.

David Lederman was instrumental in the development of an implantable artificial heart.

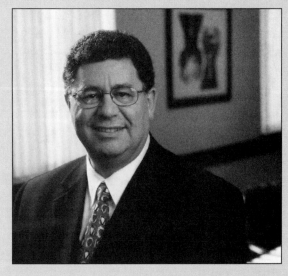

The development of the AbioCor has also resulted in several spin-off products useful to surgeons in general. One is diagnosis support software that determines the mortality risk of a particular patient group. Other developments sound like something out of *Star Trek*.

> 'We have also developed methods to transfer energy from outside the body to the inside, and to relay information from the inside to the outside, and beam it anywhere in the world without wires,' said Lederman. 'In addition, we have developed technologies for performing virtual surgery in advance of implanting an AbioCor. Some of these also have applicability to other fields outside of cardiology.'[100]

When seventy-one-year-old Tom Christerson, the second AbioCor recipient, came home from the hospital, he expected a few close friends would be there to greet him. Instead, it seemed the whole town of Central City, Kentucky, showed up. Signs on marquees and banners proclaiming "Welcome Home, Tom" were all over town. Future artificial heart recipients probably will not get such an elaborate homecoming—artificial hearts will become a routine treatment. "Nowhere else will the dependence of life on technology and the machine be more apparent," said Jarvik in 1981. "If the artificial heart is ever to achieve its objective, it must be more than a pump. It must be more than functional, reliable, and dependable. It must be forgettable."[101]

Financing the Future

Financial growth in a company whose main function is research and development is difficult. Abiomed started with grant money for research and some individual investment. The company's long-term goal was always the development of an artificial heart. Much of the funding for that invention came from sales of Abiomed's first product, the BVS 2000, a biventricular support system. The sales of the BVS have continued to fund the AbioCor clinical trials in the United States and Europe. Those sales will also

Living with an Artificial Heart

Life is pretty much back to normal for seventy-one-year-old Tom Christerson since he got out of the hospital and returned home to Central City, Kentucky. He spends his mornings talking local politics and sports and telling jokes with his "buddies" at a downtown coffee shop. Then he heads over to the barbershop. "I've talked to the barbers to see what's going on around town. They know everything. If you don't believe me, just ask them," Christerson was quoted as saying in a June 2002 Jewish Hospital press release.

About the only difference in his routine now is that he carries a red pack of batteries wherever he goes. "I'll live with it the rest of my life," Christerson says of the battery pack. "I guess I'll have to get me two or three different colors so I won't be carrying the same one all the time. You can get color coordinated." The batteries keep Christerson's brand new heart beating and him alive. Christerson is the second recipient of the AbioCor artificial heart. On September 13, 2001, surgeons Laman Gray and Rob Dowling replaced Christerson's heart with the AbioCor at Jewish Hospital in Louisville, Kentucky. On April 16, 2002, Christerson became the first AbioCor trial patient to return to his home.

"We couldn't be more pleased with Tom's progress," Gray was quoted as saying in the same press release. "Watching him return to his home and family has been a thrill for everyone involved in the project." Now that Christerson is at home, his surgeons are having a difficult time getting him back to the hospital for checkups. "After he was sent home, we did not get any calls," Dowling was reported as saying in the same press release. "I insist on him coming to Louisville for weekly office visits but he doesn't think he needs to be seen by a doctor."

help finance the artificial heart's journey to meet the Food and Drug Administration's rigorous standards. The FDA regulates and approves the use of all medical devices in the United States. To ensure their safety, new medical devices must meet certain standards before they can be used on the general population.

The idea of an artificial heart is attractive to many patients; for one thing, with a mechanical device, recipients do not have to worry about the problem of rejection. Gordon Milby, while perfectly happy with his transplant, has wondered about the new technology, especially since his doctors were the first to implant the AbioCor product in a human being. Since the artificial heart is still experimental and Milby was a good candidate for a transplant, his doctors did not consider it an option for him.

Heart transplants are also expensive. According to the United Network for Organ Sharing (UNOS), the cost of a heart transplant is almost $210,000 in the first year with annual costs of $15,000 thereafter. Most recipients need insurance or some other way to finance the operation even to be considered a candidate for heart transplantation. Of course, the number of donors also limits the number of transplants done. It is difficult to determine how much artificial heart implantation will cost. If artificial hearts prove dependable and the technology becomes part of mainstream medicine, chances are they will be less expensive than the clinical trials. But at least initially, artificial heart implantation will be expensive. And candidates for the new procedure must have the means to pay for it. Who will be chosen for artificial heart implantation? Will age and the general health of recipients be factors? Will mechanical hearts become permanent solutions or continue to be bridges to transplantation? These are some of the questions that need to be answered. Many organizations and individuals will want to have a voice in the debate.

NOTES

Introduction: Heartfelt Changes

1. Quoted in Robert G. Richardson, *The Scalpel and the Heart*. New York: Charles Scribner's Sons, 1970, p. 28.
2. Christiaan Barnard and Curtis Bill Pepper, *Christiaan Barnard: One Life*. Toronto, Ontario: Macmillan, 1970, p. 290.

Chapter 1: To Hold and Heal a Human Heart

3. Quoted in Jurgen Thorwald, *The Century of the Surgeon*. New York: Pantheon Books, 1956, p. 389.
4. Quoted in Richardson, *The Scalpel and the Heart*, p. 152.
5. Quoted in Richardson, *The Scalpel and the Heart*, p. 152.
6. Quoted in Richardson, *The Scalpel and the Heart*, p. 153.
7. Quoted in Richardson, *The Scalpel and the Heart*, p. 155.
8. Quoted in Richardson, *The Scalpel and the Heart*, p. 155.
9. Quoted in Lael Wertenbaker, *To Mend the Heart*. New York: Viking Press, 1980, p. 33.
10. Quoted in Wertenbaker, *To Mend the Heart*, p. 34.
11. Quoted in Wertenbaker, *To Mend the Heart*, p. 26.
12. Quoted in Wertenbaker, *To Mend the Heart*, p. 79.

Chapter 2: Open-Heart Surgery

13. Quoted in G. Wayne Miller, *King of Hearts: The True Story of the Maverick Who Pioneered Open Heart Surgery*. New York: Random House, Times Books, 2000, p. 69.
14. Quoted in Miller, *King of Hearts*, p. 108.
15. Quoted in Miller, *King of Hearts*, p. 135.
16. Quoted in Miller, *King of Hearts*, p. 192.
17. Quoted in Miller, *King of Hearts*, p. 87.

18. Quoted in Miller, *King of Hearts*, p. 168.

19. Quoted in Henry Minetree, *Cooley: The Career of a Great Heart Surgeon*. New York: Harper's Magazine Press, 1973, p. 133.

20. Quoted in Minetree, *Cooley*, p. 134.

Chapter 3: The First Transplant

21. Quoted in Minetree, *Cooley*, p. 153.

22. Quoted in Wertenbaker, *To Mend the Heart*, p. 195.

23. Quoted in Thomas Thompson, *Hearts: Of Surgeons and Transplants: Miracles and Disasters along the Cardiac Frontier*. New York: McCall, 1971, p. 12.

24. Quoted in Wertenbaker, *To Mend the Heart*, p. 203.

25. Quoted in Wertenbaker, *To Mend the Heart*, p. 195.

26. Quoted in Wertenbaker, *To Mend the Heart*, p. 187.

27. Quoted in Minetree, *Cooley*, pp. 153–154.

28. Quoted in *History of Transplantation: Thirty-Five Recollections*. Los Angeles: UCLA Tissue Typing Laboratory, 1991, p. 318.

29. Quoted in Miller, *King of Hearts*, p. 207.

30. Quoted in *History of Transplantation*, p. 441.

31. Quoted in *History of Transplantation*, p. 438.

32. Quoted in Richardson, *The Scalpel and the Heart*, p. 290.

33. Quoted in Christiaan Barnard and Curtis Bill Pepper, *Christiaan Barnard*, Toronto, Ontario: Macmillan, 1970, p. 256.

34. Quoted in Barnard and Pepper, *Christiaan Barnard*, p. 256.

35. Quoted in Barnard and Pepper, *Christiaan Barnard*, p. 256.

36. Quoted in Barnard and Pepper, *Christiaan Barnard*, p. 256.

37. Quoted in Barnard and Pepper, *Christiaan Barnard*, p. 257.

38. Quoted in *History of Transplantation*, p. 571.

39. Quoted in Barnard and Pepper, *Christiaan Barnard*, p. 295.

40. Barnard and Pepper, *Christiaan Barnard*, p. 309.

41. Quoted in *History of Transplantation*, p. 577.

42. Quoted in Wertenbaker, *To Mend the Heart*, p. 207.

43. Quoted in Miller, *King of Hearts*, p. 206.

44. Quoted in Minetree, *Cooley*, p. 153.

45. Quoted in Minetree, *Cooley*, pp. 158–59.

Chapter 4: Increasing Transplant Life Expectancy

46. Quoted in Thompson, *Hearts*, p. 12.
47. Quoted in Thompson, *Hearts*, p. 172.
48. Quoted in Thompson, *Hearts*, p. 109.
49. Quoted in Thompson, *Hearts*, p. 172.
50. Quoted in *History of Transplantation*, p. 570.
51. Quoted in Thompson, *Hearts*, p. 173.
52. Quoted in Wertenbaker, *To Mend the Heart*, p. 220.
53. Quoted in *Journal of Thoracic Cardiovascular Surgery*, "Diagnosis of Human Cardiac Allograft Rejection by Serial Cardiac Biopsy," September 1973, p. 466.
54. Quoted in Robert Finn, *Organ Transplants: Making the Most of Your Gift of Life*. Sebastopol, CA: O'Reilly and Associates, 2000, p. 136.
55. Quoted in Minetree, *Cooley*, p. 155.
56. Quoted in Thompson, *Hearts*, p. 172.
57. Quoted in Stephan Westaby, *Landmarks in Cardiac Surgery*. Oxford, UK: Isis Medical Media, 1997, p. 267.
58. Quoted in Finn, *Organ Transplants*, p. 135.
59. Walter Merrill, interview by author, Nashville, TN, June 2002.
60. Quoted in Mary Gohlke and Max Jennings, *I'll Take Tomorrow: The Story of a Courageous Woman Who Dared to Subject Herself to a Medical Experiment—The First Successful Heart-Lung Transplant*. New York: M. Evans, 1985, p. 129.
61. Quoted in Gohlke and Jennings, *I'll Take Tomorrow*, p. 132.
62. Gohlke and Jennings, *I'll Take Tomorrow*, p. 200.

Chapter 5: The Artificial Heart

63. William H. Frist, M.D., *Transplant: A Heart Surgeon's Account of the Life-and-Death Dramas of the New Medicine*. New York: Atlantic Monthly Press, 1989, p. 8.
64. Quoted in Thompson, *Hearts*, p. 211.
65. Quoted in Thompson, *Hearts*, p. 215.
66. Quoted in Thompson, *Hearts*, p. 216.

67. Quoted in Thompson, *Hearts*, p. 220.

68. Quoted in Westaby, *Landmarks in Cardiac Surgery*, p. 291.

69. Quoted in Westaby, *Landmarks in Cardiac Surgery*, p. 292.

70. Quoted in Kenneth Aaron, "Matters of the Heart," *Cornell Engineering Magazine*, Spring 2002, p. 15.

71. Quoted in "New Frontiers in Health and Technology: The AbioCor Artificial Heart," June 15, 2002. www.msnbc.com.

72. Quoted in "AbioCor Implantable Replacement Heart Procedure Performed at Jewish Hospital by University of Louisville Surgeons," July 4, 2001. www.heart pioneers.com.

73. Quoted in Newsweek/MSNBC, "New Frontiers in Health and Technology: The AbioCor Artificial Heart."

74. Quoted in Newsweek/MSNBC, "New Frontiers in Health and Technology: The AbioCor Artificial Heart."

75. Quoted in The Implantable Artificial Heart Project/ Jewish Hospital, "AbioCor Implantable Replacement Heart Procedure Performed at Jewish Hospital by University of Louisville Surgeons," July 4, 2001. www.heartpioneers.com.

Chapter 6: Now and the Future

76. Gordon E. Milby, interview by author, telephone, Louisville, KY, June 2, 2002.

77. Milby, interview.

78. Milby, interview.

79. Quoted in Finn, *Organ Transplants*, p. 278.

80. Milby, interview.

81. Milby, interview.

82. Quoted in Finn, *Organ Transplants*, p. 278.

83. Milby, interview.

84. Milby, interview.

85. Milby, interview.

86. Darla Granger, interview by author, e-mail, Louisville, KY, June 19, 2002.

87. Milby, interview.
88. Granger, interview.
89. Milby, interview.
90. Milby, interview.
91. Walter Merrill, interview by author, Nashville, TN, May 15, 2002.
92. Granger, interview.
93. Milby, interview.
94. Granger, interview.
95. Merrill, interview.
96. Merrill, interview.
97. Quoted in Underwood, "A Year Later, the Beat Goes On," *Newsweek*, June 24, 2002, p. 80.
98. Quoted in Underwood, "A Year Later, the Beat Goes On," p. 79.
99. Quoted in Steve Halasey, "Getting to the Heart of the Matter," *MX*, May/June 2002. www.devicelink.com.
100. Quoted in Halasey, *Getting to the Heart of the Matter*.
101. Quoted in Westaby, *Landmarks in Cardiac Surgery*, p. 291.

GLOSSARY

anesthesia: Numbing pain with or without the loss of consciousness for patients undergoing surgery.

antibiotic: Any drug that helps fight bacterial infection; penicillin was the first drug of this kind.

anticoagulant: A drug used to prevent the blood from clotting.

antivivisectionists: People who believe animals should not be used for experimental surgery or medical research.

aorta: Major artery that emerges from the heart.

artificial heart: A man-made device that pumps blood through the body just like a natural heart.

atrial septal defect (ASD): A hole or holes between the heart's two upper chambers.

atrium: An upper chamber of the heart.

biopsy: A procedure during which some tissue is removed from a transplanted organ to test for signs of rejection or disease.

bioptome: Device used to pinch off a small piece of tissue from a transplanted heart.

blood transfusion: The transfer of blood into a patient.

bypass surgery: A procedure in which a length of vein is used to redirect the flow of blood from a blocked artery to the heart.

cardiac: Pertaining to the heart.

cardiac arrest: Sudden stoppage of the heart.

cardiac assist device: A mechanical device attached to the heart that helps it keep beating; the most common is the left ventrical assist device or LVAD.

congenital heart defect: A problem with a heart, such as a hole between chambers that exists at birth.

cyanosis: A bluish discoloration of the skin caused by inadequate oxygen in the blood.

defibrillator: A device that electrically shocks a heart back to normal rhythm.

donor: A person whose organs are used for transplantation.

heart-lung machine: A machine that keeps a patient's blood circulating and oxygenated so that open-heart surgery can be performed.

hypothermia: Cooling the body in order to perform some kinds of surgery.

immunosuppressant: A drug that suppresses the body's immune system so that it will not reject a transplanted organ.

oxygenation: The bodily function of mixing blood with oxygen.

pacemaker: A surgically implanted device that sends electrical pulses to the heart, helping it maintain a normal rhythm.

pericardium: The protective sac surrounding the human heart.

plasma: That part of the blood remaining after all the cells have been removed; unlike whole blood, it does not have to be typed, and any patient can safely receive plasma from any donor.

pulmonary arteries: The arteries through which blood flows from the heart to the lungs.

rejection: The immune system's attempt to fight off a transplanted organ.

rheumatic fever: A complication of bacterial infection that sometimes damages the heart.

sutures: Surgeon's stitches used to close wounds or incisions.

vena cava: Either of two veins that return blood to the heart.

ventricle: A lower chamber of the heart.

ventricular fibrillation: The state the heart is said to be in when it is beating irregularly and so cannot pump blood.

ventricular septal defect (VSD): A hole or holes between the heart's two lower chambers.

FOR FURTHER READING

Books

Jeffrey R. Lueders, *Second Chances: Receiving the Gift of Life*. Shippensburg, PA: Ranged Edge Press, 2000. The author is a transplant recipient who has compiled a number of true stories from other transplant recipients and donors.

Frontiers of Medicine: Foundation for the Future. New York: Torstar Books, 1986. This book has a short section on the Jarvik 7 artificial heart, showing its impact on future developments, and explains how far medical science has come.

Periodicals

Robert Kunzig, "The Beat Goes On: Artificial Heart Transplants," *Discover*, January 2000.

Charles Piddock, "Have a Heart," *Current Science*, November 9, 2000.

Video

NOVA, "The Electric Heart." WGBH Boston Video, 1999.

Websites

www.abiomed.com. This official website of the maker of the AbioCor has the latest updates on artificial heart technology and on the clinical trials now in progress.

www.heartonlinecenter.com. This website offers a multitude of information about heart disease, patients' stories, transplantation, and the artificial heart. Virtually any question concerning the heart can be answered at this website.

www.heartpioneers.com. This website for Jewish
Hospital contains all updates on the clinical trials
and the patients and doctors who are involved in
them in Louisville, Kentucky.

Works Consulted

Books

Christiaan Barnard and Curtis Bill Pepper, *Christiaan Barnard: One Life*. Toronto, Ontario: Macmillan, 1970. This autobiography of the first surgeon to perform a heart transplant was written shortly after that historic operation. Written from Barnard's perspective, it nonetheless includes several interviews and stories from less well-known doctors and patients involved in those first few heart transplants.

Jenny Bryan and John Clarke, *Organ Farm: Pig to Human Transplants*. London: Carlton Books, 2001. This account of the recent history and latest developments in interspecies transplantation includes discussions of issues resulting from advances in medical technology.

Robert Finn, *Organ Transplants: Making the Most of Your Gift of Life*. Sebastopol, CA: O'Reilly and Associates, 2000. This book thoroughly explains the various stages, risks, and choices available to potential transplant patients.

William H. Frist, M.D., *Transplant: A Heart Surgeon's Account of the Life-and-Death Dramas of the New Medicine*. New York: Atlantic Monthly Press, 1989. Written by the first heart-transplant surgeon to be elected to the U.S. Senate, this book is slanted toward the author's political views on medical issues. However, it does provide some insight into how heart transplantation affects doctors, patients, and their families.

Bernard J. Gersh, M.D., *Mayo Clinic Heart Book*. New York: William Morrow, 2000. This reference book on all matters involving the heart includes excellent diagrams and illustrations.

Mary Gohlke and Max Jennings, *I'll Take Tomorrow: The Story of a Courageous Woman Who Dared to Subject Herself to a Medical Experiment—The First Successful Heart-Lung Transplant*. New York: M. Evans, 1985. This is a day-by-day account of the author's experience with heart-lung transplantation.

History of Transplantation: Thirty-Five Recollections. Los Angeles: UCLA Tissue Typing Laboratory, 1991. This series of articles on the milestones of cardiac surgery was written by the doctors and researchers involved.

G. Wayne Miller, *King of Hearts: The True Story of the Maverick Who Pioneered Open Heart Surgery*. New York: Random House, Times Books, 2000. This account of the medical career of Walt Lillehei not only includes interesting stories about surgeons, patients, and researchers; it tells each from the perpective of the times in which it occurred.

Henry Minetree, *Cooley: The Career of a Great Heart Surgeon*. New York: Harper's Magazine Press, 1973. Written by a former patient of Denton Cooley, this biography, although dated, is balanced and insightful.

William W. Moore, *Fighting for Life: The Story of the American Heart Association, 1911—1975*. American Heart Association, 1983. This book provides a direct history of the American Medical Association's first half century.

Richard G. Richardson, *The Scalpel and the Heart*. New York: Charles Scribner's Sons, 1970. This is a detailed history of cardiac surgery from ancient times until the first transplant.

Douglas Starr, *Blood: An Epic History of Medicine and Commerce*. New York: Knopf, 1999. This is an excellent history of how blood and blood by-products became of use in medicine, including an explanation of how a system for collecting and dispersing blood developed prior to World War II and how that aided in the development of modern cardiac surgery.

Thomas Thompson, *Hearts: Of Surgeons and Transplants: Miracles and Disasters Along the Cardiac Frontier.* New York: McCall Publishing, 1971. Though dated, this is a fascinating account of the fierce competition between surgeons during the early days of open-heart surgery and heart transplantation.

Jurgen Thorwald, *The Century of the Surgeon.* New York: Pantheon Books, 1956. This is a dated book but nonetheless gives an excellent account of the first surgery inside a human heart.

Lael Wertenbaker, *To Mend the Heart.* New York: Viking Press, 1980. Written by a patient of Dwight Harken, this volume includes exerpts from interviews with many well-known heart surgeons.

Stephan Westaby, *Landmarks in Cardiac Surgery.* Oxford, UK: Isis Medical Media, 1997. This book includes a collection of surgeon's recollections, medical journal articles, and commentary by innovators in cardiac surgery.

Periodicals

Kenneth Aaron, "Matters of the Heart," *Cornell Engineering Magazine*, Spring 2002.

"A Daughter's Last Gift," *Time*, September 5, 1994.

"Diagnosis of Human Cardiac Allograft Rejection by Serial Cardiac Biopsy," *Journal of Thoracic Cardiovascular Surgery*, September 1973.

"Doctor Finds Trial Reinforces His Faith," *Richmond Times Dispatch*, May 27, 1972.

"14 Dogs Die So She and Other Children Have a Chance to Live," *Minneapolis Tribune*, September 23, 1952, editorial page.

Stephen R. Large, "Is There a Crisis in Cardiac Transplantation?" *Lancet*, March 2, 2002.

"Lillehei's Offer to Operate on Twin Boys' Dog," Associated Press, January 3, 1969.

"Medical Definition of Death Upheld in Transplant Case," *Richmond Times Dispatch*, May 26, 1972.

Anne Underwood, "A Year Later, the Beat Goes On," *Newsweek*, June 24, 2002.

Internet Sources

HeartCenterOnline for Patients—For Your Heart Health, "For Cardiologists and Their Patients," December 11, 2001. www.heartcenteronline.com.

HeartCenterOnline for Patients—For Your Heart Health, "Patient Story," June 23, 2002. www.heartcenter online.com.

The Implantable Artificial Heart Project/Jewish Hospital, "AbioCor Implantable Replacement Heart Procedure Performed at Jewish Hospital by University of Louisville Surgeons," July 4, 2001. www.heartpioneers.com.

The Implantable Artificial Heart Project/Jewish Hospital, "First Patient Enrolled in AbioCor Trial Dies," November 30, 2001. www.heartpioneers.com.

The Implantable Artificial Heart Project/Jewish Hospital, "Tom Christerson Enjoys Everyday Life in Central City," June 18, 2002. www.heartpioneers.com.

Newsweek/MSNBC, "New Frontiers in Health and Technology: The AbioCor Artificial Heart," June 15, 2002. www.msnbc.com.

INDEX

PICTURE CREDITS

ABOUT THE AUTHOR

Among writer Nancy Hoffman's books are *West Virginia*, *South Carolina*, and *Eleanor Roosevelt and the Arthurdale Experiment*. She lives in Nashville, Tennessee, with her husband, daughters Eva and Chloe, one old dog, and a young cat.